MEDITATION
AND ITS PRACTICE

MEDITATION
AND ITS PRACTICE

Swami Rama

The Himalayan Institute Press
Honesdale, Pennsylvania

The Himalayan Institute Press
RR 1, Box 405
Honesdale, PA 18431 USA

Cover design by Robert Aulicino

The paper used in this publication meets the minimum
requirements of the American National Standard for
Information Sciences—Permanence of Paper for Printed
Library Materials, ANSI Z39.48-1984.

ISBN 0-89389-153-3

CONTENTS

INTRODUCTION

IT WAS JULY, 1973, and on a hill overlooking a small lake, a tent had been set up to provide shelter from rain and bright sun. More than a hundred people were gathered to listen to a series of talks by Swami Rama in the relaxed surroundings of central Minnesota farmland. He sat on a low platform, facing the length of the tent. The grassy floor of the shelter was filled with blankets, carpets, and cushions for those sitting in front of him. Because the day was warm, the canvas at the sides had been raised, and a light breeze drifted through. The timeless setting seemed an ideal complement to this accomplished teacher's words about yoga.

Through the intervening years the ideas Swami Rama expressed then have become familiar, but on that day they were new and challenging. "You are a citizen of two worlds," he began, "the world within and the world without. To be a successful person you will need to understand how to build a bridge between these two worlds. Extreme views are not helpful to the world, nor are they helpful in your own life. It is best to gain control of your thoughts, sensations, emotions, and urges." With these words he initiated the idea of working with one's self.

"Control does not mean stopping these things entirely, or over-indulging," he continued. "Control means balance. To achieve it, calm down the parts of the mind that are running so fast. You will need to rest the entirety of your mind, and for that you should learn a new way of knowing yourself. That method of inner knowing is called meditation." And with this simple introduction he began to describe the meditative process.

This was not the first time I had heard Swami Rama lecture on meditation. We had met eight months earlier at a seminar exploring the relationship between meditation and biofeedback. During the course of the seminar he spoke with me individually in a small room off the side of the main hall. When I sat down with him, a low coffee table separated us in the narrow space, and on the table was an EEG record—my own brain waves—prepared that day by seminar staff on a portable machine. He glanced at it as we talked.

"Do you meditate?" he asked.

"Not really," I replied, although I had tried on a number of occasions. Somehow I felt that my rather unorganized attempts did not constitute the answer "Yes."

"You should learn to meditate!" he responded. Soon he had gotten me started, and I left the weekend dedicated both to the goals of meditation and to an elementary technique for learning to do it. I joined a small class of his students to continue my training.

In those early years information about meditation came from a variety of sources—mainly books, articles, and class handouts prepared under Swami Rama's guidance. In addition, a few experienced teachers served as guides. As a result, a good deal of note-taking and sharing took place, and students frequently revised their method of meditation as new techniques were introduced. In addition, general concepts about meditation underwent a continual shaping process. "What *is* meditation, after all?" we seemed to be asking.

Swami Rama frequently referred to meditation as a channeling of consciousness. By this, of course, he did not mean psychic channeling. "Like the banks of a river," he said, "meditation channels awareness to be aware of itself. As with other actions you perform, meditation is a systematic process. When you understand the process, it becomes more reliable and leads to deeper experiences."

The method he taught follows the plan described by the great Indian teacher Patanjali. This approach to meditation is organized so that it focuses first on the body, next the breath, then the senses, and finally the mind. "Do not try to skip steps," he would advise. "No jumping! Follow the plan in a systematic way and it will bear fruit in its own time. If you are performing the method correctly, then it cannot fail to help you."

Discussions about practice techniques often shifted to the focus of concentration. During lectures in Nepal in 1984, Swami Rama came back to this subject many times. He reminded students that mental identification with the thoughts, forms, and names of experiences in the outer world is a habit that is difficult to break. The mind returns to these mental constructs from the moment it awakens in the morning. It becomes bound by them.

"The task of a teacher is to help bring the mind out of old grooves by giving it a new focus," he explained, and then he pondered aloud about what that new focus in meditation should be. "A picture of a teacher? The name of a loved one, or an abstract concept? In each case the mind will forget the purpose and turn outward again. But mantras," he said, "are sounds with no corresponding outer object. These vibrations create a form, but the form is not external to you. Realizing the meaning of a mantra is a matter of *becoming*. Through listening to the mantra, the many small and disturbing waves of the mind will become quiet and will be drawn into the harmony of your concentration. Then you will be able to accomplish immense, wonderful things with your life."

Swami Rama was acutely aware of the tendency to let our thoughts drift in meditation. Sometimes he approached this problem with humor, describing the puppy-like expressions of those fantasizing about pleasures and the furrowed brows of those lost in worry. But he rarely missed the opportunity of reminding students to remain alert. "Do not meditate for the purpose of dwelling on the unconscious mind. Do it to form a channel for the presence of the Atman—the indwelling Self of all," he said. "Do not brood."

In India, two decades after his Minnesota lectures, Swami Rama continued to provide the same systematic training as in the early years. "Practice regularly every day," he reminded students sitting with him near his ashram along the banks of the Ganges. "Make your ego travel toward the center of consciousness. Know that you are peace, happiness, and bliss. Freedom is your essential nature. Experience this again and again so that it becomes assimilated." Then, turning thoughtful, he added, "In this journey there is no loss of existence. There is only coming and going from this visible world. Birth is a sort of arrival, and death is a departure. You are here for a time. Meditate and you will grasp the reality of this."

Meditation and Its Practice is an introduction to a way of understanding life's journey and the mysteries of existence. The message is timeless. The techniques are systematic. Its subject, of course, is your own self-transformation. I hope that in the course of reading this your interest in meditation will blossom, because with this practice, despite the occasional blows delivered by daily affairs, life does become tranquil.

Rolf Sovik, Psy.D.

PREFACE

THIS BOOK WAS WRITTEN to provide a clear, systematic manual of the basic techniques of meditation. It is meant to give you a progressive, step-by-step approach that is practical rather than philosophical or theoretical. It also introduces the most important practices used in preparing yourself for meditation. These preliminary practices will greatly enhance the quality of your meditation.

For thousands of years, the science of meditation has been studied and practiced by aspirants who sought to make their lives more serene, creative, and fulfilling. Meditation will give you the capacity to improve your health, your relationships, and the skillfulness with which you perform your activities. This is because meditation can do something no other technique can accomplish—it introduces you to yourself on all levels and finally leads you to the center of consciousness within, from which consciousness flows through all the tributaries of life. This center or higher self is called *Atman*.

The seeker's aspirations are fulfilled when they become fully aware of Atman, the inner dweller, and no longer identify with the objects of the mind and the world. When this occurs, the aspirant becomes established in the realm of Atman, a blissful inner state called *samadhi*. After attaining this state, all questions are answered and all problems are resolved.

While the basic practices are simple to learn, you will find that the more consistently you practice, the more fully you will experience the benefits. At first you may notice simple changes, such as increased calmness and resistance to stress, but as you progress you will notice deeper and more significant developments within yourself. This inward journey is very pleasant, provided you are persistent and practice regularly.

In fact, the practical science of meditation is so profound and interesting that you may find yourself intrigued and challenged by other aspects of yoga, including *asanas* (physical yoga postures), *pranayama* (the science of breath), issues related to improving your health, and the underlying philosophy and psychology of meditation.

May you enjoy and benefit from the process you have begun.

CHAPTER ONE

WHAT IS MEDITATION?

THE WORD *MEDITATION* is used in a variety of ways, so there is a good deal of confusion about what precisely meditation is and how to practice it. Some people mistakenly use the word *meditate* to mean thinking or contemplating; others use it to refer to daydreaming or fantasizing. However, meditation is not any of these, but a different and distinct process, which is important to fully understand.

Meditation is a specific technique for resting the mind and attaining a state of consciousness that is totally different from the normal waking state. In meditation, you are fully awake and alert, but your mind is not focused on the external world or the events taking place around you. Neither is your mind asleep, dreaming, or fantasizing. Instead, it is clear, relaxed, and inwardly focused.

The root of the word *meditation* is similar to that for *medical* or *medicate*. The root of all these words implies the sense of "attending to" or "paying attention to" something. In meditation, you pay attention to dimensions of yourself which are seldom known—your own deepest, innermost levels. These deeper levels are more profound than the processes of thinking, analyzing, daydreaming, or experiencing emotions or memories. Meditation involves a type of inner attention that is quiet, concentrated, and at the same time relaxed. There is nothing difficult or strenuous about creating this inner attention; in fact, you will find that meditation is a process that is restful for the mind. In the beginning, the greatest difficulty is that the mind has never been trained to create this inner attention.

In every society all over the world, people are educated in the skills needed to survive and function in their culture—how to talk, think, work, and investigate the objects and experiences of the external world. We learn sciences such as biology, ecology, and chemistry in order to understand the world we live in, but no one—in any school, college, or university—teaches us to understand or attend to our own inner dimensions. We merely learn to assimilate the goals, fashions, and values of our society without really knowing ourselves first, within and without. This leaves us ignorant of ourselves and dependent on the advice and suggestions of others.

Meditation is a different, subtle, and precise approach. It is the simple technique of learning how to pay attention to and understand the various levels of yourself—the body, the breath, and the mind. As time progresses, you may find that you enjoy the positive results of meditation—increased joyfulness, clarity, and awareness—as much as you enjoy the relief you will experience from releasing the physical, nervous, and mental symptoms of stress.

This meditation manual offers systematic guidance in the practice of meditation and will answer the most common questions about getting started. With these techniques you can continue on your own for some time. Ultimately, there are stages in meditation where external guidance from an experienced meditator is necessary and beneficial. However, this book will help you with the most important basic practices. You will find that you do not need to do anything physically different or demanding, that your meditation does not require you to adopt any strange or foreign habits, and that you do not have to be able to meditate for long or extended periods of time in order to progress and observe the benefits. You will find that you enjoy the practice of meditation. Your body will be more relaxed, your mind will become more creative and focused, and you may even notice significant improvements in your health and relationships.

Meditation is therapeutic from the beginning. It helps relax muscular tension and the autonomic nervous system, and provides freedom from mental stress. A person of meditation attains a tranquil mind, and this helps the immune system by limiting its reaction to stress and strain. You will find that even a few days' sincere effort will help you control your appetites—and even reactions such as anger, to a certain degree. Meditation will also decrease your need for sleep and will energize your body and mind. This is a result we have observed with students from all walks of life.

Those who are writers, poets, and thinkers often express interest in becoming more creative and developing their intuition, the finest and most evolved of all aspects of knowledge. Meditation is a systematic way of enhancing our innate talents in daily life.

Meditation also has an important influence on health. In the modern world, most diseases can be classified to some degree as psychosomatic, having their origin in or being influenced by thoughts and emotions. Recently, scientists have begun to recognize that these kinds of diseases cannot really be cured merely by the conventional methods of orthodox medicine or psychotherapy, because if disease originates in your mind and your emotional reactions, how can an external therapy alone restore your health? If you rely only on external remedies and do not seek to understand your own mind and emotions, you may merely become dependent on a therapist or physician for help. In contrast, the method of meditation makes people self-reliant and helps them attain the inner strength necessary to deal more effectively with all of life's problems.

Meditation as a Process

In the process of meditation, we ask the mind to let go of its tendencies to think, analyze, remember, solve problems, and focus on the events of the past or on our expectations about the future. We help the mind to slow down its rapid series of thoughts and feelings, and to replace that mental activity with inner awareness and attention. Thus, meditation is not thinking about problems or analyzing situations. It is not fantasizing or daydreaming or letting the mind wander aimlessly. Meditation is not having an internal conversation or argument with ourselves or intensifying the thinking process. Meditation is simply a quiet, effortless, one-pointed focus of attention and awareness.

In meditation, we try to let go of the many mental distractions, preoccupations, and fleeting thoughts and associations of our normal waking experience. We do this, not by trying to make the mind empty, which is impossible anyway, but by allowing the mind to focus on one subtle element or object, which leads the attention further inward. By giving ourselves one internal focus of attention, we help the mind stop other stressful mental processes, such as worrying, planning, thinking, and reasoning.

The student of meditation may be given an internal device to help concentrate the mind. Most often, a sound is used in this manner, although sometimes a visual image for concentration is suggested. The sound or image may be either external or subtle, according to the frame of mind of the aspirant. Sounds which are used to concentrate the mind in meditation are called mantras. Mantras have powerful effects on the mental level.

A mantra may be a word, a phrase, a set of sounds, or simply a syllable. Concentrating on a mantra helps students let go of other useless, distracting mental processes, and allows them to go deeper inside themselves. Many different kinds of mantras are used throughout the world, including ones such as *Om, Amen,* and *Shalom,* and all have the goal of helping to focus the mind. In this book we will introduce a basic mantra for your practice. Using that mantra regularly will be most beneficial.

In all great spiritual traditions of the world, ancient and modern, there is some system of pronouncing such a syllable, sound, or set of words which acts like a mantra. This is a great and profound science, and those who are competent in this inner science can lead students on the path. The preliminaries practiced by aspirants are simple and easy and can be done without the guidance of a teacher, but when an aspirant begins to deal with the mind, an appropriate mantra will be necessary. Using a mantra given by a teacher adept in the meditative tradition can produce powerful and effective results.

Meditative texts and scriptures speak extensively on this subject. Patanjali, the codifier of yoga science, says that the mantra is a representative of the innermost source of consciousness. Therefore, it becomes a bridge between the mortal and immortal parts of life. When the body, breath, and conscious mind separate from the unconscious mind and individual soul at the time of death, the mantra that the meditator had been consciously remembering continues to create impressions in the unconscious. These impressions are powerful motivators which help the aspirant during this period of transition. With the help of the mantra, it becomes easier for a person to make the unknown voyage.

Mantra is the support and focal point given to the mind. Teachers choose a mantra according to the aspirant's state of mind and the extent of the aspirant's burning desire to uncover the innermost truth.

Just as there are many different paths one can take to climb a mountain, there are also a variety of seemingly different meditation techniques. Yet all have the same goal—achieving a state of inner concentration, calmness, and serenity. Any practice that helps you achieve this is beneficial. Many valid techniques exist, so there is really no difference between one type of authentic meditation and another, as long as they have the goal of helping you attain inner stillness and focus.

Sometimes people become caught up in comparing meditation methods or arguing about which tradition or teacher is "best." Good meditation teachers recognize and respect the universality of meditation and do not foster self-serving or cultish distinctions about their techniques. Meditation is a beneficial and fruitful way of exploring the inner dimensions and fathoming all levels of life systematically. It is positive and valuable, as long as teachers do not become egotistical and try to claim a style of meditation as their own or insist that their technique is superior.

In the beginning, the aspirant does not have the clarity of mind necessary to discover or understand the correct method of meditation, and may be influenced by teachers who promote their own type of meditation. Sadly, some of these teachers are dishonest and do not even really practice meditation themselves. Many students waste valuable time seeking an authentic meditative discipline, jumping from one teacher to another. After spending much time, energy, and money on this quest they may become disappointed and frustrated and finally stop making a sincere effort. In the Himalayan tradition, we sometimes say that if there is any such thing as sin in this world, a prime example would be a teacher's confusing or misleading sincere students.

If we observe life clearly, we realize that from our childhood onward, we have only been educated to examine and verify things in the external world and that no one has actually taught us how to look within, find within, and verify within. Therefore, we remain strangers to ourselves, while trying to get to know others. This lack of self-understanding is why our relationships don't seem to work successfully, and why confusion and disappointment prevail in our life.

Very little of the mind is cultivated by our formal educational system. The part of the mind which dreams and sleeps, the vast realm of the unconscious which is the reservoir of all our experiences, remains unknown and undisciplined; it is not subject to any control. It is true that the whole of the body is in the mind, but the whole of the mind is not in the body. There is no other method to truly develop control over the totality of the mind except the practice of meditation.

We are taught how to move and behave in the outer world, but we are never taught how to be still and examine what is within ourselves. At the same time, learning to be calm and still should not be made a ceremony or religious ritual; it is a universal requirement of the human body. When we learn to sit still, we attain a kind of joy that is inexplicable. The highest of all joys that can ever be experienced by a human being can be attained through meditation. All the other joys in the world are momentary, but the joy of meditation is immense and everlasting. This is not an exaggeration; it is simply stating a truth supported by the long line of great sages, both those who renounced the world and attained truth, and those who continued living in the world yet remained unaffected by it.

The mind has a tendency to dwell in the grooves of its old habit patterns, and to imagine experiences which may occur in the future. The mind does not really know how to be in the present, here and now. Only meditation teaches us to fully experience the now, which is our link with the eternal. When, with the help of meditative techniques, the mind is made one-pointed and inward, it attains the power of penetrating into the deeper levels of our being. Then the mind does not create any distractions or deviations, and fully achieves the power of concentration, which is a prerequisite for meditation. How fortunate are those who become aware of this fact and begin to meditate. Even more fortunate are those who continue to meditate, and the most fortunate are those few who have determined that meditation is the top priority in their life, and practice it regularly.

To begin this path, understand clearly what meditation is, select a practice that is comfortable for you, and do it consistently for some time, every day if possible, and at the same time every day. In the modern world, however, students tend to become impatient easily and do a practice for only a brief period of time before they give up, concluding that there is no value or authenticity to the technique. This is like a child who plants a tulip bulb and is frustrated because he sees no flowers in a week. You will definitely experience progress if you meditate regularly—it is not possible for you to fail to progress if you do the practice.

At first you may see progress in terms of immediate physical relaxation and emotional calmness. Later you may notice other, more subtle signs. Some of the most important benefits of meditation make themselves known gradually over time, and are not as dramatic or easily observed. Persist in your meditation and you will experience progress. Later we will discuss how to assess your progress and when to move on to the next step.

Before we conclude this discussion, we will try to clarify the distinctions between some other mental processes which are often confused with meditation.

What Meditation Is Not

Meditation is not contemplation or thinking. Contemplation, especially the contemplation of inspiring concepts or ideals such as truth, peace, and love can be helpful, but it is different than the process of meditation. In contemplation, you engage your mind in inquiry into a concept, and ask the mind to consider the meaning and value of a certain idea. In the system of meditation, contemplation is considered a separate practice, although one that also may be useful at times. When you engage in meditation, you do not ask the mind to think about any concept, but rather to go beyond this level of mental activity.

Meditation is not hypnosis or autosuggestion. In hypnosis, a suggestion is made to the mind, either by another person or yourself. Such a suggestion may take the form "You are getting sleepy (or relaxed)." Thus, in hypnosis there is an attempt to program, manipulate, or control the content of the mind, to make the mind believe something helpful or make it think in an ordered, particular way. Sometimes such suggestions can have useful effects, as the power of suggestion is powerful. Unfortunately, negative suggestions also commonly have destructive effects on various levels of our being.

In meditation, you do not make any attempt to give the mind a direct suggestion or to control the mind. You simply observe the mind and let it become quiet and calm, allowing your mantra to lead you deeper within, exploring and experiencing the deeper levels of your being. In the meditative traditions, a practice such as hypnosis is thought to have some potential liabilities. For example, it may create conflict in the mind because of subtle resistance to the external influence used in the suggestion. Practices such as hypnosis or autosuggestion may have some therapeutic effects, but it is important not to confuse them with meditation. The sages say that meditation is actually the opposite of hypnosis; it is a state of clarity and freedom from suggestion or outside influence.

Meditation is not religion. Meditation is not some strange or foreign practice that requires you to alter your beliefs, reject your culture, or change your religion. Meditation is not a religion at all, but rather a practical, scientific, and systematic technique for knowing yourself on all levels. Meditation does not belong to any culture or religion of the world, but is a pure and simple method of exploring the inner dimensions of life and finally establishing oneself in one's own essential nature. Some schools call this innate nature *samadhi*, others *nirvana;* some call it perfection or enlightenment. It can also be called Christ-consciousness. Such words and labels do not matter at all. The system of meditation promotes inner spirituality, not any particular religion.

Some people promote practices they call meditation, but which are really a mingling of meditation with religion or other cultural values. This makes students anxious that meditation might interfere with their religious faith, or that they will have to give up their own culture and take up another culture's customs. This is definitely not the case. Religion teaches people what to believe, but meditation teaches you how to experience directly for yourself. There is no conflict between these two systems. Worship is a part of religion, as is prayer, which is a dialogue with the Divine. Certainly you can be both a religious person who prays and a meditator who uses the techniques of meditation, but it is not necessary either to belong to or to reject an orthodox religion in order to meditate. Meditation should be practiced as a pure technique, in a systematic, orderly way.

In order to meditate, you will need to learn:
- How to relax the body.
- How to sit in a comfortable, steady position for meditation.
- How to make your breathing process serene.
- How to calmly witness the objects traveling in the train of your mind.
- How to inspect the quality of your thoughts and learn to promote those which are positive and helpful to your growth.

• How to remain centered and undisturbed in any situation, whether you judge it to be bad or good.

This book will systematically cover all these points, so that your meditation becomes enjoyable, deep, and effective. If you practice meditation with a clear understanding of what it is, and with the appropriate techniques and attitude, you will find it refreshing and energizing. Now that you understand this basic background material, you are ready to go on to the next step—preparing to meditate.

Chapter Two

Preparation for Meditation

THE MOST IMPORTANT and most often overlooked step in meditation is that of preparation. Without the appropriate preparation, physical, mental, or emotional distractions will create obstacles that prevent your meditation from becoming deep or profound. And while the physical body does not itself produce the meditative state or help you meditate, physical problems or discomforts can certainly create barriers or distractions in your meditation.

The most common physical problems are: illness; physical discomfort caused by tension or an inability to relax so that you can sit comfortably; fatigue or drowsiness; being physically agitated, jittery, or restless from the day's stressful events; and problems with food—either being hungry or having eaten excessively. Most of these common physical barriers to meditation can be eliminated by becoming increasingly aware of how you manage your lifestyle. Of course it's true that prevention is better than cure. While you can certainly continue to meditate if you have a cold or other minor physical problems, you will probably find that the discomfort, pain, or inability to concentrate that accompany any severe illness is a real obstacle to meditation. Fortunately, meditation tends to make you more sensitive to many physical processes, helping you prevent illness by becoming more attuned to what your body needs in order to stay well.

Recommendations for how to remove these problems will be given in this book. Special practices will be provided for the removal of physical tension and stress. In addition, the issues of food and adequate sleep, and how they affect meditation practice, will be addressed later in this chapter.

Some Basic Guidelines

An advanced meditator can sit in meditation almost anywhere. For most of us, however, paying attention to some basic guidelines will greatly increase the ease of meditation. There are no special or unusual prerequisites for meditation—you can meditate at home, in the country, in the city, at the shore, or in the mountains. It does help, however, if the place you have chosen for meditation is relatively quiet, peaceful, uncluttered, and restful.

Ideally, a small corner of your room or home can be set aside as your meditation space. This should have good air circulation and not be stuffy, musty, or uncomfortable. A clean, quiet place is all you need. It is best if this space is apart from the main "busy-ness" of your life, away from the kitchen, television, or telephone, and not where others will interrupt you. Similarly, it may be wise to avoid a place like an office, which may have associations that distract you mentally. Choose a quiet, pleasant corner or area of a room. It is not recommended that you meditate on your bed because your mental associations with sleep may make it hard to stay alert and awake there. Whether you sit on a chair or on the floor as described in the next chapter, it helps to select a special place and reserve it for meditation.

Meditation can be done any time, night or day, but traditionally the best times—when the environment is most conducive to meditation—are said to be early morning and late evening, when the world around you begins to quiet down and you are not likely to be interrupted by others. You may be naturally freshest and more alert either in the morning or the evening, so that may be your own best time to meditate. However, your schedule and your personal responsibilities will also have a great impact on when you can meditate.

If you are a parent with small children, it will probably be easiest to meditate when the children are in bed. At first, try to select one or two brief periods (5 to 15 minutes) when you can meditate without inconveniencing others, being disturbed, ignoring your duties, or feeling rushed or preoccupied by other tasks. The easiest way to adjust your routine may be to rise a little earlier in the morning or to meditate just prior to bed at night.

You will find that your meditation progresses most rapidly if you create a regular time you can reserve for meditation every day. Establishing this habit and making it a reliable, predictable part of your schedule is extremely beneficial in deepening practice. Even if your schedule shifts from day to day, try to find a suitable time and be as consistent and regular at that time as possible. This helps to eliminate the mental resistance caused by laziness and the tendency to procrastinate.

First step: cleansing

First, prepare the body physically. Meditation is easiest when the body feels fresh, comfortable, relaxed, and clean. Taking a shower or even simply washing your face, hands, and feet will help to give you a fresher feeling. In the morning, your body will feel most comfortable meditating if you empty your bladder and bowels before you prepare for meditation.

Second step: stretching

Some people find that their body feels stiff and achy after sleeping all night. In such cases a warm bath and gentle stretching exercises will help to prepare the body to sit in meditation.

The hatha yoga *asanas* (postures) were specifically developed to maintain physical health and to help the body become strong and supple enough to sit comfortably in meditation. Some basic postures that are beneficial in preparing for meditation are taught in *Yoga: Mastering the Basics*. Ideally, however, asanas should be learned personally from a qualified instructor.

Stretching and limbering the back and legs can significantly increase your comfort in meditation. Even a few minutes of stretching or yoga asanas can create a vast improvement in the quality of your meditative experience. Unlike strenuous aerobic exercise, these hatha yoga postures will not tire you or overly activate your body. Instead, they gently energize you, relax your muscles, help you let go of mental stress, and focus your concentration. In the beginning, consider spending at least 5 to 10 minutes stretching and preparing the body before meditation.

Third step: relaxing

After you complete your stretching exercises you will find it beneficial to do a brief relaxation practice. Lie comfortably, with your back flat on the floor or on a padded surface. Use a thin cushion under your head. Cover your body with a sheet or thin shawl. Lie with your arms slightly separated from the body, palms turned up. Place your legs a comfortable distance apart. Make sure that your body weight is evenly distributed and that you are not twisting or leaning to either side. Your head should also be centered and not tilted in either direction, as this will create tension in the neck. This relaxation position is called the corpse posture, *shavasana,* because you are lying completely still and very relaxed. Let your eyes remain gently closed and take several minutes to become aware of your breath, exhaling and inhaling through your nostrils slowly and smoothly, without any interruptions or pauses.

Lying in this posture, you can lead yourself through a brief relaxation exercise, systematically paying attention to each major muscle group, moving progressively through your body. A complete description of this practice is given in the appendix. You may also be interested in using a guided relaxation tape. Relaxation practices should be brief, and should not last longer than about 10 minutes. You will need to ask your mind to remain alert, because for many people the tendency for the mind to drift off to sleep will become evident.

Fourth step: calming the mind and nervous system

The breathing process is a powerful variable, which has an enormous impact on the tension level of your body, as well

as on the calmness and clarity of your mind. Before meditation, special yogic breathing practices are done in a meditative
sitting posture in order to help create a calm mental state
conducive to an inward focus, concentration, and serenity.
Some students may initially feel a little resistant to spending
time on these practices. However, once you have done
them, you will notice that they aid immeasurably in deepening meditation. The breathing process and its role in emotional balance and mental clarity are fascinating. Later we
will describe several specific breathing exercises that have a
vital and beneficial effect on meditation.

Fifth step: sitting in meditation

After you complete your breathing practice, you are ready
to meditate. Sit in your meditative posture (a variety of such
postures will be described in the next chapter) and simply
allow your mind to become aware of your own mantra, or
of the universal mantra *so hum,* a sound that is coordinated
with the breath in a special way. As you exhale, mentally hear
the sound *hum;* as you inhale, mentally hear the sound *so.*

Let your breath lengthen and become smooth. Sit quietly
and allow your mind to focus on the mantra. Continue to
sit comfortably in your meditation posture, letting your
mind become quiet and centered. You may sit for as long as
is comfortable or for whatever time you have available on
that occasion. When you are ready to end your meditation,
first bring your awareness back to the breath and then to the
body. Make the transition from the state of internal awareness to external awareness a gradual one by gently covering
your eyes with cupped hands and then opening your eyes to
look first at the palms of your hands. What happens with
the mind in meditation, and how you work with the mind,
will be discussed in detail in the following chapter.

Thus, the order of practice is as follows: first, bathing or preparing; second, stretching exercises or yoga postures; third, relaxation exercise; fourth, breathing practices; and finally, meditation itself.

Before we complete this general discussion, there are other important issues related to the preparation for meditation that deserve special attention.

Other Factors Influencing Meditation

Yoga psychology describes four "primitive fountains," the four primary drives that motivate us all. These are the urges for food, sex, sleep, and self-preservation. Each of these urges needs to be skillfully managed if our meditation is to progress. Imbalances in these four urges have physical and emotional consequences that may interfere significantly with the ability to concentrate and meditate.

From the meditative perspective, a healthy diet is composed chiefly of fresh, simple food that is not overcooked, overprocessed, or greasy, nor excessively roasted or toasted. These tend to cause digestive problems which interfere with meditation. Fresh, simple, natural food that is nutritious and easy to digest is most beneficial.

The atmosphere in which food is eaten should also be pleasant and joyous. In our modern society husbands, wives, and children are busy away from home all day; they only have the opportunity to come together and discuss the day's events at the dining room table. But this time should not be made unpleasant or negative; the family should have the understanding that no unpleasant discussions should occur at this time. Cheerfulness is traditionally said to be the greatest of all physicians. Those who are aware of this important secret of good health know that while they are eating they should be happy. A pleasant, cheerful state of mind has a powerful effect on the efficiency of the digestive system and the secretion of the endocrine glands.

Many diseases and physical problems can be prevented once we understand the functioning of our body and its language. When good food is eaten in pleasant surroundings and in a good mood, our body produces saliva and gastric juices effectively, aiding in the digestion of food. Eating in a depressed mood, or during heated, negative discussions, can create digestive disorders.

All food should be thoroughly chewed. It is best to fully enjoy your food by eating slowly and taking time to taste it. To promote good digestion, there should also be an adequate amount of liquid in the food. Fresh fruits and salads should also be a part of your diet.

Overeating should be avoided because of the many problems it causes. After a meal, rinse and clean the mouth and teeth, and then allow the digestive system to rest, without snacking between meals. Food should always be taken at least four hours before meditation, sex, or sleep. Eating food and then immediately retiring to bed is not a healthy habit.

The process of digestion and your body's reaction to foods can have powerful influences on your meditation. In fact, one cannot really meditate for three to four hours after eating a large meal. For this reason, the early morning hours are ideal for meditation. Your body should have finished digesting the previous day's meals and should feel light and fresh. In the evening, you will find that if you eat a late, heavy dinner, you will have to wait until fairly late at night to be able to really concentrate or meditate.

Obviously, the kinds of foods you eat will cause a range of different results. A light, fresh meal of vegetables, fruits, and grains may not take much time to digest, while a heavy feast with rich, fatty foods may take hours. Further, you will probably find yourself increasingly aware that certain foods help you feel clear, relaxed, and centered while you meditate. Conversely, foods may also cause a variety of interferences. Some foods will make you restless, agitated, and tense, creating a jittery feeling. Others may make you drowsy or sluggish, creating so much heaviness you can barely remain awake in meditation. As you continue to experiment with your reaction to foods, you will become increasingly aware of how particular foods affect your mental state.

It is not necessary that you become a vegetarian in order to meditate. In fact, if you don't know how to create a well-balanced vegetarian diet, an abrupt change in your eating patterns could cause you some significant difficulties. So be gentle with yourself. A well-balanced vegetarian diet, with fresh fruit, dairy products, and well-cooked vegetables, grains, and legumes, may be helpful, particularly if it is low in fat. If you decide to make changes in your diet, you may want to first consult a resource book, such as *Transition to Vegetarianism*, to guide your efforts.

The effects of food and beverages on the depth of meditation are powerful. As you continue your meditation practice, your attraction to food (as well as many other things) may gradually evolve in a healthier direction, and you may become increasingly skilled in noticing the subtle effects of what you eat or drink. Many people who initially drink large amounts of coffee, tea, or other caffeinated beverages begin to notice that doing so creates physical and mental agitation. The topic of food and its effect on meditation and consciousness is so important that it actually deserves an entire book. Some basic suggestions:

• Before you meditate, allow 3 to 4 hours after eating a large meal.

• Be aware of what you have eaten and how it affects your meditation later in the day.

• Select fresh, wholesome, easy-to-digest foods which promote the clarity and calmness vital to meditation.

In addition, you will soon begin to notice that alcohol and any other mood or mind-altering substances you have been using may cause significant interference in your meditation. No one who genuinely understands meditation thinks that drugs are helpful in attaining a meditative state, because drugs agitate the body and distract the mind through their toxic effects. Alcohol can create a sluggish, drowsy, dull state that is an obstacle to meditation. Most people find that their attraction to these substances decreases as they become increasingly drawn to the tranquility of meditation.

Sleep, like food, is a physical process that may also have a significant influence on your meditation. Too little sleep will make you drowsy and you could have difficulty remaining awake during meditation. However, too much sleep can be equally disruptive, making you sluggish, groggy, or unable to concentrate.

Sleep is a fascinating process, which is interesting to examine as you learn to meditate. Generally speaking, as your meditation deepens your need for sleep decreases, because meditation creates a deep, restful state for both body and mind.

As you progress in your meditative practice and it becomes more important to you, you will want to find ways to meditate at a time that allows you to be alert and fresh. Increasingly, it becomes a priority to plan your life so that food, sleep, and other activities support rather than interfere with your meditative practice.

CHAPTER THREE

MEDITATIVE POSTURES

MEDITATION IS A SIMPLE TECHNIQUE almost everyone can enjoy. As we said earlier, to meditate, simply sit quietly and comfortably in a relaxed and steady position. Still the body, make the breathing process serene, and then allow the mind to become quiet and focused. We need to discuss these three aspects of the meditative process in more detail: first, how to position the body so it is at ease, yet remains steady; next, why it is important to cultivate a serene manner of breathing and how to accomplish that; and finally, how to still the mind and make it one-pointed and focused, so that meditation itself can take place. These three stages move awareness from the most external physical level to the most subtle inner level. We will begin by considering the position of the body in the process of meditation.

The requirements for a good meditation posture are that it be still, steady, relaxed, and comfortable. If the body moves, sways, twitches, or aches, it will distract you from meditation. Some people have the misconception that to meditate, you must sit in a complicated, cross-legged position called the Lotus Pose. Fortunately, this is not accurate. There is actually only one important prerequisite for a good meditation posture—it must allow you to keep the head, neck, and trunk of the body aligned so that you can breathe freely and diaphragmatically.

In all the meditative postures the head and neck should be centered, so that the neck is not twisted or turned to either side, nor is the head held too far forward. The head should be supported by the neck, and held directly over the shoulders without creating tension in either the neck or shoulders. Face forward with your eyes gently closed. Simply allow your eyes to close; don't squeeze them shut or create any pressure in your eyes.

Unfortunately, some people have been told to force their gaze upward at a point on their forehead. This creates strain in the eye muscles and may even produce a headache. There are some yogic practices that involve specific gazes, but they are not used during meditation. Simply let all your facial muscles relax. Your mouth should also be gently closed, without any tension in the jaw. All breathing is done through the nostrils.

In all the meditative positions, your shoulders and arms should be relaxed and allowed to rest gently on your knees. Your arms should be so completely relaxed that if someone were to pick up your hand, your arm would be limp. You can gently join the thumb and index finger in a position called the "finger lock" (see photograph at right). This *mudra* (gesture) creates a circle, which you can think of symbolically as a small circuit that recycles energy within.

Sitting Positions for Meditation

There are many positions that allow you to keep the spine aligned and to sit comfortably without twisting your legs or creating any discomfort. In fact, the arms and legs are not really

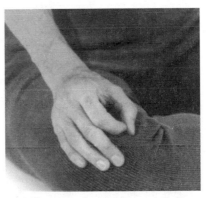

Finger lock (*jñana mudra*)

important in meditation. What is important is that the spine be correctly aligned. The easiest way to accomplish this is a posture called the friendship pose, *maitri asana* (see photograph on p. 26).

In the friendship pose, you sit comfortably on a chair or bench, with your feet flat on the floor and your hands resting gently in your lap. The friendship pose can be used by anyone, even those who are not flexible or who aren't comfortable sitting on the floor. This posture allows you to begin the process of meditation without creating any difficulty for the body.

The easy pose (sukhasana)

If you are somewhat flexible, you may want to begin sitting in an alternative position called the easy pose, *sukhasana* (see photographs on p. 27). In the easy pose, you sit in a simple, cross-legged position. As you can see in the photograph, each foot is placed on the floor under the opposite knee, and the knees rest gently on the opposite feet. Sit on a thick, folded blanket, so that your knees and ankles do not receive too much pressure.

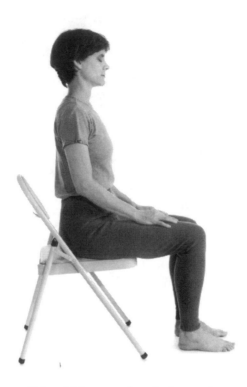

Friendship pose (*maitri asana*)

If your legs are not flexible or your thigh muscles are tight, you may find that your knees are fairly far off the floor. A cushion or another folded blanket placed beneath your buttocks will help you. Doing several warm-up stretching postures will also be beneficial in developing greater flexibility, so you can sit more comfortably in this position. Whatever position you select, practice it regularly and avoid frequent attempts at new postures. If you work regularly with developing one sitting pose, it will become comfortable and steady over time.

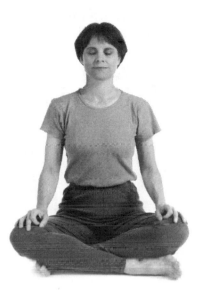

Easy pose (*sukhasana*)

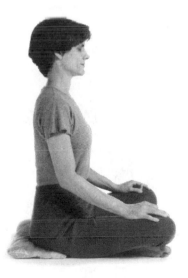

Making your sitting posture more comfortable

The auspicious pose (swastikasana)

The auspicious pose, *swastikasana* (see photograph below), offers several advantages for those who can sit in it comfortably. If your legs are fairly flexible, you may actually find it more comfortable than the easy pose for longer periods of meditation. Because the position has a different, wider foundation, it distributes your body's weight more evenly over the floor, and is somewhat steadier and less likely to lead to swaying or other bodily movements.

As you can see in the photograph, in the auspicious pose the knees rest directly on the floor rather than on the feet. One advantage of this posture for some students is that the ankle bones receive less pressure.

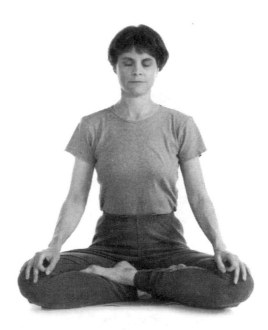

Auspicious pose (*swastikasana*)

To assume *swastikasana,* begin by sitting comfortably on your meditation seat, and then bend the left leg at the knee and place the left foot alongside the right thigh. The sole or bottom of the left foot should be flat against the inside of the right thigh. Next, bend the right knee and gently place the right foot on the left calf, with the bottom of the foot against the left thigh. Gently place the outside surface of the right foot between the thigh and the back of the left calf, tucking in the toes. Finally, use your hand to gently bring the toes of your left foot up between the right thigh and calf, so that the big toe is now visible. This creates a symmetrical and stable posture, which is quite helpful for meditation. While the above description may sound complicated, you will find that if you follow the directions, it is not difficult.

Other Considerations

For some beginning students, the auspicious pose may not be comfortable initially because they lack flexibility in their legs. You can certainly sit in any individual variation of a cross-legged pose that allows you to be steady and keep your body still without jerkiness or swaying, or you may begin, as we said earlier, with the friendship pose. This vital point is worth repeating: It is more important to keep the head, neck, and trunk correctly positioned, so that the spine is aligned, than to put your legs in any particular position.

Some students become competitive about advanced positions, assuming them before they are properly prepared. As a result, they may sit incorrectly because they hunch their shoulders over, creating a curve in their spine. This is a bad habit to develop, as it will create physical discomfort and obstruct your breathing. It will also interfere with the subtle energy channels in your body, which become increasingly important in deeper meditation.

Modern people tend to have poor posture because of bad habits they developed as children while walking and sitting. Because of this, the muscles which are meant to support the spinal column are underdeveloped, and the spine tends to curve with age, distorting the body. When you first begin sitting in meditation, you may notice that your back muscles are weak and that after a few minutes of sitting you tend to slump forward.

Actually, this problem can be solved rather quickly if you begin paying attention to your posture throughout the day while sitting, standing, and walking. Adjust your posture when you notice that you are slouching. In this way, your back muscles will begin to do their job appropriately. Certain hatha yoga postures—the cobra, boat, bow, and child's pose—are also helpful in strengthening your back muscles so that they can support the spinal column.

Some students with poor posture ask if they can do their meditation leaning against a wall for support. In the beginning you can do this to develop a correctly aligned posture or to check your alignment, but it is not good to remain dependent on an external support. From the start it is best to work attentively and consistently with your posture. Ask a friend to check your posture, or do it yourself by looking sideways in a mirror. If your spinal column is correctly aligned, you will not feel the knobs of the spinal vertebrae jutting out while you run your hand up your back.

Other Meditation Postures

Several other positions are often considered appropriate for meditation. We will briefly discuss some of the issues relating to these postures.

The thunderbolt pose (Zen sitting position)

Some people who have had hip or knee problems may have difficulty sitting in the cross-legged positions. They may have heard they should sit on their legs with the hips over the ankles in a position known as the thunderbolt pose.

Unfortunately, trying to sit directly on the floor in this position places excessive strain on the feet and ankles, and may cause problems with the muscles or nerves. If you prefer this kind of position, it is better to use one of the wooden "Zen benches" that are commercially available. You then sit directly on the bench or seat, removing your full weight from your ankles and feet. There are other drawbacks to this position: the posture tends to be less stable for longer meditations, and is more likely to allow the body to sway or shift sideways. For some students, however, physical limitations may make this pose their best option.

The accomplished pose (siddhasana)

Traditionally, the accomplished pose (also called the adept's pose) was taught to certain advanced students, although it is not recommended as a posture for general use (see photograph on p. 32). This is because, like the lotus pose, the accomplished pose requires the ability to put the body into a particular position which is only helpful if it is done precisely and correctly. If you do not have the ability to sit in the posture perfectly yet comfortably, you will not get its benefits and can even create problems for yourself.

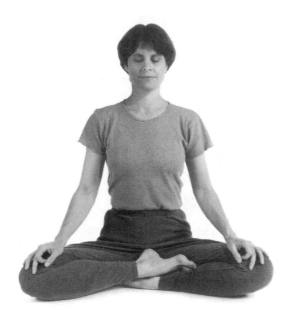

Accomplished pose (*siddhasana*)

Siddhasana was never a position recommended for beginners or for those who intended to live in the world.

However, those who are adepts, or who have decided to lead a deep meditative life, should gradually learn to sit in this posture. Those who have decided to attain samadhi, particularly, should practice this posture during meditation. Advanced students of meditation form the habit of sitting in *siddhasana* in order to accomplish their goal. When an advanced student can sit in this pose for more than three hours at a time, without any pain, then *asana siddhi* (perfection of posture) is acquired. However, it is not necessary for beginners, who are not yet ready, to put their body in a position in which they will be uncomfortable. Trying to sit in a position for which one is unprepared can result in injuries due to pulled muscles or ligaments.

To assume *siddhasana,* place the left heel at the perineum (the region between the anus and the genitals) after applying the root lock. (This is done by contracting the anal sphincter muscles, pulling them in.) Now place the other heel at the pubic bone above the organ of generation. Arrange the feet and legs so that the ankles are in one line, or touch each other. Place the toes of the right foot between the left thigh and calf so that only the big toe is visible, and gently pull up the toes of the left foot between the right thigh and calf so that the big toe is visible. Place the hands on the knees.

To repeat, we do not recommend this posture, except to those who learn it under direct personal guidance, because it can create problems for a student if done incorrectly. Traditionally, this position was taught to males who intended to live as monks. However, it is false to think that men alone can sit in this posture: women meditators and nuns do practice this pose.

The lotus pose (padmasana)

Like the accomplished pose, the lotus pose is generally not recommended for meditation, because unless it is applied precisely, it is not beneficial. Almost no one can sit absolutely correctly and comfortably in this posture, especially since it is difficult to perform other important practices called *bandhas* (locks) while in this position.

Padmasana is closely associated with yoga in the popular imagination, but advanced yogis and meditators actually use only *siddhasana.* The lotus flower is a symbol for yogic life, which involves living in the world yet remaining unaffected by it, just as the lotus lives in the mud, yet floats its exquisite blossoms above the surface of the water.

Presently, the lotus pose is taught as an exercise to make the lower extremities limber and supple, rather than being used for actual meditation, because for most students sitting in this position is too uncomfortable to allow concentration. Since pain and discomfort prevent most students from reaching a meditative state, we recommend that students sit in another posture which is steady and also comfortable.

In summary, for most students, using one of the first three positions described here will allow them to make the most consistent progress. Cultivate one position and regularly use it for meditation. If you do this, you will find that the posture becomes increasingly comfortable, steady, and still.

Suggestions for Making Sitting Positions More Comfortable

You will probably find it easiest to sit on the floor if you use a folded blanket to provide padding over the area. Then, use a thick cushion or pillow placed directly under your buttocks and hips, lifting that part of your body off the floor by three to four inches. Elevating the buttocks in this manner relieves much of the pressure on the hip joints and knees. You may be amazed at the difference it makes. Using a thick cushion under your buttocks will also make it easier to keep your spine correctly aligned. Your meditation seat should be firm, but not too hard or shaky. The seat should not be so high that it disturbs your body position.

As you become more flexible and comfortable, you may find that you can use a thinner cushion and even eventually sit flat on the floor. However, it is important to keep the spine aligned and not allow it to curve, disturbing your posture. At first some people find it difficult to maintain this alignment without a thick cushion. Be patient in developing your sitting posture. You will find that your body will gradually become more flexible and you will eventually be able to sit for longer periods more comfortably.

Stretching exercises and hatha yoga asanas can be beneficial in helping you to make your body more flexible and comfortable in meditation. For further information or help with hatha practices, you may want to take a hatha yoga class or refer to *Yoga: Mastering the Basics*.

It is not recommended that you meditate while lying down. There are several reasons for this. One of the most important is that most people rapidly fall asleep in a reclining position, or have difficulty maintaining any alertness or awareness. Obviously, if you are dozing or asleep, you won't be able to meditate.

Actually, there is also a more subtle reason. At deeper levels of meditation it is important to be able to sit with the spine correctly aligned, since this allows a certain type of subtle energy to move upward through the body. This interesting topic is dealt with in detail in several advanced books on meditation, such as *Path of Fire and Light*.

CHAPTER FOUR

MEDITATION, MIND, AND MANTRA

ONCE YOU KNOW how to sit in a meditative posture, you will probably wonder what to do mentally; how exactly does one begin to meditate? People wonder if they should think specific thoughts, or if they should try to make the mind completely empty, or if they should just allow the mind to drift and let associations flow into the mind. Actually, meditation does not involve any of these alternatives.

Thinking is a different process than meditating and, as we noted earlier, even contemplating on an inspiring ideal, such as peace, is a different process. Trying to make anything happen in the mind in meditation is fruitless—you will simply become frustrated, because the mind seems to fight attempts to control it. The motivation to achieve some specific state is actually of little help in meditation. It's usually better not to create pressure for yourself about how your meditation should be or what to expect. Ironically, the less you fight with yourself or force yourself to meditate, the more you will relax and reach greater stillness, which is what progress in meditation really means.

Similarly, it will not work to try to make the mind empty. By its very nature the mind changes, processes memories, makes associations, and takes in new information. In fact, usually the only time the mind becomes even somewhat still is in the state of deep, dreamless sleep. The rest of the time it tends to drift like a sailboat without an anchor.

Because of these mental processes, many meditative traditions seek to quiet and focus the mind by allowing it to concentrate on one object or stimulus at a time. Thus, the goal is not to make the mind empty, but rather to quiet the mind by giving it a single focus. In many meditative traditions, a word, phrase, sound, or symbol is used to give the mind this one-pointed focus on which to concentrate. Some meditative disciplines favor the use of visual symbols, while in our tradition the emphasis is on the use of a mantra—a word, sound, or set of words that one uses to give the mind an object of concentration.

Concentration is an important prerequisite for meditation. When we use the word *concentration,* sometimes we mean the sense of effort necessary to think carefully or analyze, a process which may even sound a little stressful. However, the word *concentration,* as we use it here, certainly does not imply effort, tension, or mental strain—it simply means focused attention. This is in contrast to a scattered, distracted state of mind. Concentration means an alert, yet relaxed, focus of attention, and if you are relaxed and comfortable, this kind of concentration should not be difficult. When you cannot concentrate, it means your ability to choose to direct the flow of your mind has been impaired.

Many yogic techniques aid in the development of concentration, and some of these will be discussed in detail later in this book. For now, it is important simply to understand that concentration is a prelude to meditation.

Many meditative traditions use mantras. As we pointed out earlier, the words *Amen, Shalom,* and *Om* are all mantras. In our tradition, mantras are heard mentally, coming from within, rather than spoken out loud and heard with the physical ear. The science of mantra is a unique discipline and area of study; in the yoga tradition these sounds are not used lightly or trivially. Mantras are special sounds that have particular characteristics and effects. Not just any word can be a mantra.

Sounds vibrating in themselves have no literal meaning and are known only as vibrations. When they affect material substances, these vibrations create forms and their forms have names. Yet, actually, all forms and names result from the pure vibrations of sound. There are particular sounds which vibrate in silence and are very powerful and beneficial in their effect on the entire human being. In ancient times sages, who devoted their lives to meditation, heard these sounds within, which are now used as mantras. These special sounds have different effects on different aspirants; receiving a mantra from an authentic teacher is like receiving a prescription given by a physician.

There are numerous sounds, syllables, or words which are used as mantras, and each has effects on different levels of the personality. These effects of the mantra are conveyed through an inner feeling generated within the meditator. This feeling is not the result of the literal translation of a mantra, but arises from the pure vibration of the sounds themselves. Aspirants allow the word or mantra given by the teacher to become part of their life.

Many students try to coordinate the mantra with their inhalation and exhalation; however, not all mantras are intended to be coordinated with the breath. There are even a few mantras which can create jerks or a rhythm in the breath that could be injurious to the motion of the lungs, and thus, to the heart and brain. Therefore, do not try to coordinate all mantras with the breath. The sounds that are used with the breath include *So Hum, Om,* and *Omkar,* but other mantras should not be coordinated with the breath.

Mantras should only be imparted by experienced, competent teachers. Using mantras from books is not at all helpful. The technique of how to use a particular mantra is imparted directly to the student by the teacher. Only teachers thoroughly trained in an authentic tradition understand how to convey and appropriately use a particular mantra If a teacher is unqualified and cannot transmit this proper understanding to the student, the benefits of the practice may not occur. Ultimately, mantra is a powerful tool—a compact prayer. Constant prayer creates awareness, and constant awareness leads to self-realization.

In the modern world, the science of mantra is difficult to understand because we have come to believe that only words, not apparently meaningless sounds, have truth or value. Mantras operate at a deeper level. A mantra has an effect because of its qualities of vibration and sound rather than because of its literal meaning. Meaningfulness is a property of words, yet the goal in meditation is not to deal with meanings, using the analytical part of the mind, but instead to experience ourselves at much deeper levels. The entire science of meditation and mantra is fascinating, and interested readers may want to further pursue their study of the use of mantra in meditation. See, for example, *The Power of Mantra and the Mystery of Initiation.*

All sounds have certain qualities. Some are soothing, others are energizing. The purpose of the sounds we call mantras is to help us focus the mind so we can attain a deeper experience than that created by thought alone. While many traditions use mantras, in our tradition we encourage students to begin by using the natural and universal sound *so hum.* This is a general practice which can be used by most students. *So hum* is used in a particular way. As you sit quietly in meditation, calm and quiet the breath. Let your breath become slow, smooth, and regular. Then, allow your mind to mentally hear the sound *so hum.* Mentally hear the first part, the softer sound, *so,* with the inhalation, and the second part, *hum,* during the exhalation. Simply sit quietly and let the sound repeat itself with each breath, allowing the flow of breath to remain serene.

There are several important points to note here. The first is that the mantra is only heard mentally; it is not repeated aloud or with the mouth and vocal apparatus. As you continue to allow the mantra to repeat itself, you may find that the mind will create fewer distractions. In our normal waking awareness, mental activity usually consists of chains of associations or related thoughts and feelings. Some of these are intentional or goal-oriented, while others simply seem to pop up in our minds. In meditation, as we allow this mental noise to quiet itself, we keep the mind focused on the sound *so hum.* You will note that other thoughts do enter your mind, and your awareness will shift to other issues. When this occurs, allow yourself to "witness" or nonjudgmentally observe the associations in the mind, and then gently bring your awareness back to *so hum.*

It is important not to create a mental tug-of-war during this process. When thoughts arise in the mind, simply witness them and bring the mind back to the sound *so hum*. In this way your meditation will deepen most easily. It is not helpful to engage in mental arguments or become angry or judgmental with yourself about mental distractions. Such emotional reactions consume even more energy. Thoughts will continue to arise, but most will dissipate if you witness them in a neutral way, without creating an internal conflict. This process of witnessing is different from suppressing or repressing thoughts, because you are not seeking to keep certain kinds of thoughts from coming to consciousness. When they do occur, however, notice their existence without dwelling on them or intensifying them.

It is important to remember that not all mantras can be coordinated with the breath in quite this way. In fact, you actually want to first calm and relax the breath and then let go of that awareness. Your goal is not to keep on paying attention to the process of breathing itself. Most mantras will not coordinate with the exhalation/inhalation rhythm, and if you try to force the mantra to follow the waves of your breath, you will create a distraction for yourself and disrupt your breathing. However, *so hum* meditation can be used effectively as a practice by almost everyone.

It is equally important to understand that as your meditation progresses, you may want to expand your mantra practice by receiving a personal mantra from a qualified teacher. These practices should be given personally by someone who is qualified to do so; mantra practices should not be self-prescribed from books. Mantras do have powerful effects, but in order for a student to obtain the benefits, the practice must be appropriate for the student's level of experience. This can be determined by a competent teacher who is trained to impart these techniques.

The mantra *so hum,* like all mantras, has an effect because of the way sound affects us. While we might literally translate *so hum* as "I am That" ("My inner self is united with universal consciousness"), it is not due to the meaning of these words that the mantra has an impact. It is the effect of the sound that helps the mind become still and eventually go beyond sound, to experience the silence within.

Sometimes students who come from religious backgrounds worry that their mantra comes from a foreign tradition. As we said earlier, mantra as a technique is used in many traditions, but mantra meditation itself is not a religious process. A qualified teacher, however, will be able to help you develop a practice that does not create resistance or a sense of conflict within your mind. *So hum* does not belong to any religion. It is a pure technique that helps to quiet and focus the mind.

At first, when you are able to sit in meditation for only a few minutes, you will find that your mind may be somewhat distracted and noisy. However, as you create greater mental and physical stillness by paying attention to the foods you eat, the breathing process, and the kinds of mental influences you take in, you will find that mental noise and distractibility tend to decrease. As you gradually increase the length of your meditation, you may also notice that your mind tends to slow down and become quieter as the session of meditation progresses. In the chapter on breathing we will specifically address the link between mental serenity and the breathing process.

To sum up, the actual technique of meditation is simple. Sit quietly, allow the breath to become even, and allow the

mind to become calm and quiet. Attend to the mantra arising within yourself, and keep bringing your mind back to
the mantra when it wanders. While this process is not hard
to describe, you may find it challenging to accomplish, because the mind is agile and tends to maintain a certain level
of internal chatter. Often we are not aware of how noisy the
mind is until we begin the practice of meditation. Our goal
is to allow the noise to still itself. In part, we do this by letting go of things which create conflict or mental turmoil.

The issue of progress in meditation becomes an important question for many people. In most of our activities, we
can reassure ourselves that we are making progress by observing the external aspects of our behavior. We notice that
we can go farther, faster, or for longer periods of time.
Meditation, however, presents a new situation: we cannot
simply equate sitting for longer periods with meaningful
progress. Sometimes we may sit for a long time, but our
mind is scattered, distracted, and anything but peaceful.

Because of this insecurity about progress, and uncertainty
about whether one is meditating correctly, some people become victims of a sensationalized view of meditation. They
think that if their meditation is truly going well, they should
have some dramatic mental experiences, such as perceiving
visions, lights, or colors. The simple truth is that, as meditation progresses, there should be a deepening sense of quiet
and stillness. No dramatic phenomena are required.

Some people may experience physical sensations—twinges,
twitches, or other kinds of impressions. These generally indicate that there is either tension somewhere in the body or the
presence of mental and emotional reactions, which should
not be mistaken for experiences of deeper states of consciousness. Whatever phenomenal experiences arise, students

are encouraged to let them pass and keep their attention focused on the mantra, which will slowly and gradually take them to deeper levels of their own inner nature.

As your meditation practice becomes deeper, you will also probably become aware that certain types of experiences lead to distractions. If you observe the kinds of experiences which preoccupy your mind, you will generally find that pleasant, happy feelings seldom create problems, although negative emotions or cravings can demand so much attention that all your mind wants to do is obsess about them.

At this point, you begin to notice that the kinds of thoughts you have, and the experiences you seek out, create either inner peace or inner chaos. You become increasingly aware of what kinds of experiences facilitate or disrupt your meditation later in the day. This opens up a whole new area for observation and spiritual development. You begin trying to live your life in such a way that you do not constantly create unpleasant experiences that dominate your mind or tie up your mental energy. Cultivating experiences that lead to harmony and stillness is a valuable aspect of preparing for meditation.

In this sense, the meditator becomes an internal explorer and investigator, who is studying the internal reactions and processes of the mind on both the conscious and unconscious levels. The meditator is an interior researcher whose findings help bring out levels of creative intelligence which can be useful in the external world. Meditation helps one to fully know and understand all the capacities of the mind—memory, concentration, emotion, reasoning, and intuition. Those who meditate begin to understand how to coordinate, balance, and enhance these capacities, using them to their fullest potential. Then, through the practice of meditation, they go beyond the usual states of mind into the highest realms of consciousness.

As you begin to observe the beneficial effects of meditation on your body, your mind, and the whole of your personality, you may become interested in the deeper practices and techniques that form the more advanced part of the system of meditation. If you sincerely and conscientiously do your meditation practice, you will definitely perceive many gradual changes. Don't give up out of impatience or laziness. You will make steady progress if you continue your practice.

CHAPTER FIVE

BREATHING PRACTICES

BREATH AWARENESS is an essential part of the practice of meditation, yet it is often misunderstood or underestimated by beginners. The most well-established schools of meditation teach breath awareness before introducing students to advanced techniques of meditation. In the practice of meditation, students first learn to still their body, having become aware of physical twitches, tremors, and movements. Next, they learn the breathing techniques, which help them become aware that they can develop conscious control over the body, breath, and mind.

All of the yogic breathing exercises are part of the science of pranayama, which helps the student regulate the motion of the lungs. Without such regulation, the respiratory system, heart, brain, and autonomic nervous system do not function in a coordinated way, and disturbances in these physical processes limit progress in meditation. Understanding the role of pranayama practices is important. *Prana* means "the first unit of energy," a subtler level of energy within the human personality that is the link between the body and mind. Pranayama practices allow the student to channel and balance the flow of this subtle energy, which is responsible for the well-being and coordination of all the body's functions.

Whenever any emotional strain is experienced in life, we can immediately observe its effect on the body by noticing how the breathing process changes. When we are shocked or surprised, we may unconsciously hold our breath; when we are anxious or stressed, our breathing becomes rapid and shallow. Our breath reflects the state of our mind at all times.

When life is chronically stressful, we may develop the habit of rapid, shallow breathing, which further disturbs our body and agitates our mind. In fact, the more rapid and shallow the breath, the more difficult it is to think clearly or allow the mind to become quiet. Thus, the breathing process can have a powerful effect on the depth of our meditation.

Learning about the science of breath and how to work with our own breath is vital for anyone who wants to learn advanced techniques of meditation. Once we have learned to sit in a quiet place in a comfortable, steady posture, and gross physical tension or tremors are no longer a source of disturbance, we may notice four irregularities in the breath. These are: shallowness of breath, jerks in the breath, noisy breathing, and extended pauses between inhalation and exhalation. These problems create disturbances in the mind and prevent concentration. They need to be eliminated to allow meditation to deepen.

In the ancient tradition of meditation, teachers did not impart the advanced techniques of meditation until they had determined that the student had attained stillness of the body and serenity of the breath. Sitting still is important— the less movement, the more steady the mind will be. All of the movements, gestures, tremors, and twitchings of the body are caused by an untrained mind. When we observe our behavior, we find that there is not a single act or gesture that is independent of the mind. The mind moves first, then the body moves, and the more the body moves, the more the mind is dissipated.

The Science of Breath

The breath is the bridge between the body and the mind. Inhalation and exhalation are like two sentries in the city of life, and their behavior changes instantly according to our thoughts and emotions. Inhalation and exhalation are the vehicles through which prana—the vital force—travels in the body.

The sages observed that the breath is a kind of barometer, which registers the conditions of the mind and the influence of the external environment on the body. For example, the breath can warn us of impending illness. Patanjali, the codifier of yoga science, explains that we can coordinate and quiet the mind by practicing the science of breath. According to our school of meditation, after we have established a still and comfortable posture, breath awareness is the next important step. Breath awareness allows us to create an undisturbed and joyous mind. When the breath begins to flow freely and smoothly through both nostrils, the mind attains a state of joy and calmness. Such a mental condition is necessary to allow the mind to travel into deeper levels of consciousness, for if the mind is not brought to a state of joy it cannot remain steady, and an unsteady mind is not fit for meditation.

When we start to meditate on the breath, we can observe the four defects in its flow that were mentioned earlier: shallowness, jerkiness, noise, and (that which disturbs us the most) an extended pause between inhalation and exhalation. Much has been said in the meditative scriptures about these obstructions, but practice makes us increasingly aware of the importance of dealing with them. When we begin to meditate on the flow of the breath, we notice that jerks and pauses correspond with mental distractions. Therefore it is important to learn pranayama practices that allow us to eliminate these problems.

Those who do not want to do pranayama exercises can still practice meditation, but without breath awareness a deep state of meditation is impossible. The breath and the mind are interdependent. If the breath is irregular and jerky, the mind is dissipated. After we attain steadiness in our posture, breath awareness is the next natural step in the movement toward tranquillity. It strengthens the mind and makes it much easier to turn our attention inward. It is advisable for beginners to start by becoming aware of the breath. This is the simplest, most natural, and most essential step for attaining a deeper state of meditation.

Those students who are prepared for an advanced meditation technique realize the importance of breath awareness. When the mind begins to follow the flow of the breath, we become aware of a deeper reality within, for there is a link between our innermost self and the center of the cosmos, which supplies life energy to all living creatures. As long as the body receives the vital force called prana through the breath, the body/mind relationship is sustained. When this connection is disrupted, the conscious mind fails, and the body is separated from the inner unit of life. This separation is called death.

Breath awareness enables us to experience deeper levels of

consciousness that are normally beyond the reach of the conscious mind. The truth is that we cannot develop a deeper state of consciousness without working systematically with the breath. The first step in this process is the development of breath awareness.

Most of the time we are totally unaware of the breathing process. The goal after establishing our physical posture is to turn our attention to the flow of the breath, noticing how it flows, its quality of smoothness, from where in the body the breath seems to arise, and finally, the rhythm of the breath itself.

For example, you may notice that you breathe with your mouth slightly open or that your breathing is rapid, shallow, and irregular, or that your breath makes a soft wheezing sound. The goal is to reestablish the body's natural respiratory pattern, which is even, diaphragmatic breathing. In this breathing pattern all inhalations and exhalations flow through the nostrils rather than the mouth, and the entire process is silent. If you are breathing rapidly and shallowly, you are probably chest breathing, which means that you are not allowing your breaths to be full and complete and you are probably only using part of your lungs' natural capacity. When you establish diaphragmatic breathing, you allow the lungs to expand fully with the inhalation and to be emptied more completely on the exhalation.

When you breathe evenly and diaphragmatically, breathing becomes more efficient; you will breathe more slowly because each breath carries more air and life-force. However, it is impossible to breathe diaphragmatically unless the head, neck, and trunk of the body are correctly aligned. To understand this it may be helpful to look at the diagram on page 51.

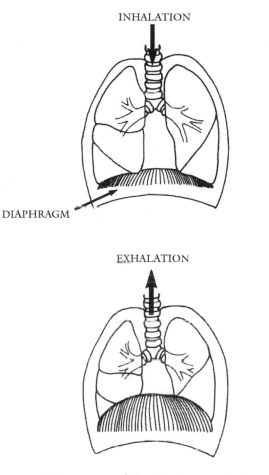

INHALATION

DIAPHRAGM

EXHALATION

**Movement of the diaphragm during
inhalation and exhalation.**

Your lungs are actually elastic and expansive, and when
they are efficiently filled, their capacity is far greater than
when we breathe shallowly, as in chest breathing. The lungs
are separated from the lower abdominal cavity by a horizon-
tal muscle called the diaphragm, which moves up and down

within the torso. As the diaphragm moves up, the lungs are emptied; as the diaphragm comes down, the lungs are allowed to fill more completely. You cannot observe the diaphragm directly, but when you breathe diaphragmatically you may notice that the lower ribs flair out slightly on inhalation, and the abdominal area may also move out a bit. On exhalation, the abdominal area moves back in toward the spinal column.

If your posture is poor and your spine is curved, you will be unable to breathe freely and will unconsciously constrict the movement of diaphragmatic breathing, resulting in rapid, shallow breaths. This is one reason why your sitting posture is so important. If your spine is poorly aligned, you cannot breathe freely, and when the breathing process is disturbed, the mind will become agitated.

The first step in practicing diaphragmatic breathing is to become aware of your posture, and to learn to be comfortable in an erect, correctly aligned position. This allows diaphragmatic breathing to develop. Then you begin to notice whether your exhalations and inhalations are equal in length. While there are some breathing exercises that intentionally alter the length of the exhalations or inhalations, most people do this unconsciously, and this is damaging to the body.

One way to reestablish an even pattern is to mentally count the length of the inhalation and exhalation, allowing them to become equal. However, in counting the duration of the breath, you may notice that there is a tendency to pause slightly as you think each number. A better way to do this is to exhale as if you were breathing down to your toes and inhale up to the crown of your head. It is important to keep the entire process even and smooth in flow, without any jerkiness or irregularity. At the conclusion of the smooth exhalation, you begin another inhalation, and continue on in this manner. If you begin to pay attention to the breathing process when you are not meditating, you can learn to correct this problem, and then when you meditate, the breath will be naturally smooth and even.

The next point is also important. Many people unconsciously hold the breath between exhalation and inhalation. This is an extremely bad habit because it tenses the body, disrupts the normal breathing rhythm, creates an imbalance in the nervous system, and, by throwing off the healthy respiratory rhythm, is said to be damaging to the heart. Eliminating this unconscious tendency to pause or hold the breath is an important goal. The entire breathing process should be smooth and natural, without any breathlessness, gasping, or feeling of being forced.

When the breath is smooth and there is no force or constriction, then it will also naturally be silent. Noisy breath means either that you are using force to breathe or that there is some obstruction or congestion in your respiratory passages.

The breathing process has become fine and subtle when your breathing is deep, even, and diaphragmatic; when the lengths of your exhalations and inhalations are equal; when your breath is silent; and, finally, when there is no pause between the inhalation and the exhalation and between the exhalation and inhalation. When this occurs, meditation can go to a deeper level.

Because the stress and strain of daily life has distorted your natural breathing rhythms, you have to consciously reestablish this normal process. At first this will require attention both during meditation and during the day's other activities. Although most students do not want to be told this, you should actually plan to spend four weeks consciously attending to the breath—learning how to breathe diaphragmatically before you turn your attention to other aspects of meditation.

Perfecting diaphragmatic breathing

There are several techniques which will help you to perfect your diaphragmatic breathing. First, lie on your back on the floor in the relaxation pose known as the corpse posture, *shavasana*. If you place one hand on the chest and the other on the abdomen at about the navel area, it will be easy for you to tell whether you are breathing diaphragmatically because you will feel a gentle movement at the navel as the abdomen rises with inhalation and falls with exhalation. If you are breathing diaphragmatically, you will not feel much movement in the chest.

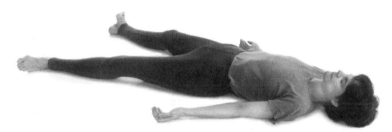

Corpse pose (*shavasana*)

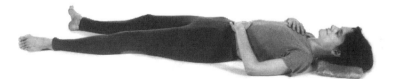

Establishing diaphragmatic breathing

You can also do a breath awareness practice in this position using a sandbag weighing about 6 to 10 pounds, which is placed across the abdomen. Simply lie in the corpse posture and pay attention to the movement of your abdominal area. This exercise will also gently strengthen your diaphragm muscle.

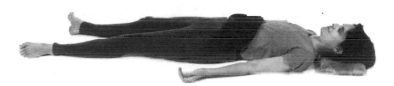

Using a sandbag

Lying on your stomach in the crocodile pose will also help you become aware of your diaphragmatic breathing. In the crocodile pose, you lie face down with your feet pointing outward. Rest your forehead on your crossed forearms and breathe deeply. In this position it will be easy for you to feel the movement of the abdomen against the floor. Breathing and relaxing in this posture for 5 to 10 minutes twice a day, morning and evening, can help you to make diaphragmatic breathing a habit. Once you can comfortably maintain diaphragmatic breathing while lying down, and have learned to maintain it in your daily activities, it will become normal to breathe this way while sitting upright in meditation.

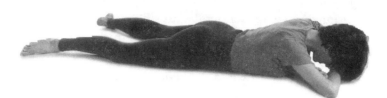

Crocodile pose (*makarasana*)

Two-to-one breathing exercise

When you have mastered diaphragmatic breathing, you will notice that your meditation changes. There are also several other practices that will be helpful to you. Two-to-one breathing will help you to relax, eliminate waste gases from the body, and increase your stamina and endurance. You can do it while sitting or while walking, and you will find it energizing.

To do this practice, make your exhalation twice the length of your inhalation. For example, you may exhale to a count of eight, and then inhale to a count of four. Do not hold the breath; let the exhalation and inhalation flow into one another without jerks or pauses. Experiment with this exercise for 5 to 10 minutes a day for two weeks and you will notice that you feel more energetic.

Pranayama and the Nervous System

The science of pranayama is closely connected with the autonomic nervous system. Pranayama techniques are intended to help balance the functioning of the nervous system, and bring these usually involuntary processes under conscious control. They are important preparatory practices for meditation, and if you experiment with them and observe their effects, you will find that they have significant benefits: calming and relaxing the body, and stilling the mind.

Long before our modern knowledge of the nervous system was acquired, the ancient yogis were aware of the flow of prana energy through channels called *nadis*. The nadis are not the same as nerves, but are the subtler coordinates of the physical nerves. There are thousands of nadis, three of which play a particularly important role: *sushumna, ida,* and *pingala*.

Sushumna is the central channel, and corresponds to the physical spinal column. The other two nadis, ida and pingala, are associated respectively with the left and right sides of the central column. Ida and pingala originate at the base of the spine. Ida terminates in the left nostril, and pingala in the right. Normally energy flows through these two side columns in alternation. The goal of many pranayama practices is to allow pranic energy to flow upward through sushumna, which engenders a state of joy, serenity, and higher consciousness.

Modern physiological research has confirmed what the ancient yogis experienced long ago—that the predominant flow of the breath shifts back and forth between the left and right nostrils. Although the average person might be surprised to discover it, one nostril is always more open than the other; air flows more freely through it than through the other, more obstructed nostril. This more open nostril is called the active or dominant nostril, while the less open nostril is considered to be passive.

In a healthy person, this process of nostril dominance will shift about every ninety minutes to two hours, as the active and passive nostrils exchange roles. The physiological process that makes this possible is fascinating. The tissues in the nasal passage on one side engorge with blood, becoming more full, and slightly closing the airway. At the same time, the passage on the opposite side becomes more open, to allow a greater volume of air flow.

It is easy to determine which of your nostrils is active at this moment: simply exhale slowly through your nostrils, placing your fingertips in the flow of the exhalation. The side from which you feel the greater and easier volume of air flow is the active or dominant nostril at this time.

If you have difficulty perceiving a difference, you can use a small pocket mirror to do a test. Place the mirror under your nostrils and notice the vapor pattern that condenses on the glass of the mirror. One pattern is usually somewhat larger, indicating the active nostril. Even when your head is badly congested, neither side is ever really completely closed. As indicated, about every ninety minutes this pattern will shift, so if you check later, it is likely that you will notice the opposite pattern.

According to ancient yogic texts, this is just the beginning of the science of breath, *swarodaya*, an intricate and precise science that is intriguing. If your interest in this amazing subject deepens, you may want to study other texts, such as *Science of Breath* or *Path of Fire and Light*, to increase your understanding. However, to return to the main point, the goal of the pranayama practice is to develop the skill to voluntarily control the respiratory process and to create a joyful, deep state of mind that is conducive to meditation by learning to open both nostrils simultaneously. For this purpose, a series of pranayama practices are taught, one of the most important of which is called *nadi shodhanam* or alternate nostril breathing.

Alternate Nostril Breathing (Nadi Shodhanam)

There are many variations of alternate nostril breathing and each has a particular purpose. As the name implies, they

all share the process of alternating the flow of breath between the two nostrils. You will find this breathing practice
to be an effective tool for helping to calm the nervous system. It is said to purify and balance the nadis, to balance the
flow of breath in the nostrils, and to create a state of clarity
and serenity suitable for meditation. It also helps balance the
functioning of the autonomic nervous system.

As your practice of alternate nostril breathing advances,
there are more subtle and extensive variations, including
some that involve retaining the breath. In our tradition,
however, we do not encourage students to begin with breath
retention. Holding the breath should not be done unless the
student has a profound knowledge of *bandhas* (locks) and
mudras (gestures), so only advanced students are taught retention. Retention intensifies the mind's focus, and if the
mind is not serene and balanced, this may not be beneficial.

Alternate nostril breathing is a simple practice to learn. There
are three versions taught in the beginning to intermediate
stages of practice. One round of each version is diagrammed
on the following pages. Select one of these and practice it
for about two months, until it has been refined. Then other
variations may be added to your practice or substituted.
After a period of practice it is best to select one pattern for
regular daily use and not to vary this pattern unnecessarily.

Nadi shodhanam is done sitting upright in a meditative
posture. It is done after asanas and relaxation, and is a
preparatory practice for meditation. It should be done at
least twice a day, morning and evening. It can also be practiced midday, but only on an empty stomach—before meals.
(Note: the midday practice pattern is determined by identi-
fying which nostril is active and which is passive at the time
of practice. See the diagrams that follow.)

Basic procedures for alternate nostril breathing

Select the variation of alternate nostril breathing you will use for your practice.

Variation I is the most refined method of practice. It is often learned first and may remain the primary practice method. It does require, however, the most frequent manipulation of the nostrils and may not be the best method for some beginners for that reason.

MORNING	MIDDAY	NIGHT
Left Right	Active Passive	Left Right
Nostril	Nostril	Nostril

↑↓3x	↑↓3x	↑↓3x
through both nostrils	through both nostrils	through both nostrils

E=Exhale   I=Inhale

Variation II is a method that is somewhat easier to remember and monitor. The alternation of the nostrils corresponds with the completion of each full breath.

MORNING	MIDDAY	NIGHT
Left Right	Active Passive	Left Right
Nostril	Nostril	Nostril

↓E ↑I	↓E ↑I	↓E ↑I
↓E ↑I	↓E ↑I	↓E ↑I
↓E ↑I	↓E ↑I	↓E ↑I
↓E ↑I	↓E ↑I	↓E ↑I
↓E ↑I	↓E ↑I	↓E ↑I
↓E ↑I	↓E ↑I	↓E ↑I

↑↓3x	↑↓3x	↑↓3x
through both	through both	through both
nostrils	nostrils	nostrils

E=Exhale   I=Inhale

Variation III requires the least amount of manipulation of the nose, and for that reason it is an easy method to learn. If the other methods prove somewhat difficult at first, this method may prove to be a good starting method.

MORNING	MIDDAY	NIGHT
Left　Right	Active　Passive	Left　Right
Nostril	Nostril	Nostril

MORNING	MIDDAY	NIGHT
↓E		
↑I		
↓E		
↑I		
↓E	↓E	↓E
↑I	↑I	↑I
	↓E	↓E
	↑I	↑I
	↓E	↓E
	↑I	↑I
↓E	↓E	↓E
↑I	↑I	↑I
↓E	↓E	↓E
↑I	↑I	↑I
↓E	↓E	↓E
↑I	↑I	↑I

↑↓3x	↑↓3x	↑↓3x
through both nostrils	through both nostrils	through both nostrils

E=Exhale　　I=Inhale

1. In a seated meditative position, check the alignment of your head, neck, and trunk, so that your spine is correctly positioned and you can breathe freely.

2. Determine whether to begin by exhaling through the right or the left nostril. The choice depends upon the time

of day and the method being used (see the diagrams).

3. Breathe diaphragmatically. In this exercise all the exhalations and inhalations should be of equal duration and should be smooth, slow, and controlled. Do not allow the breath to be forced or jerky. Allow the eyes to remain gently closed.

4. A special hand position is used to gently close the nostrils in alternation. Bring the right hand up to the nose, and fold the index and middle fingers to the palm, so that you can use the thumb to close the right nostril, and the ring finger to close the left nostril. Be sure that you are not bending over to bring the head down to your hand. Also be aware of how much pressure you use with your thumb and ring finger in closing the nostril. Very little pressure is needed. You can simply rest the thumb or finger against the side of the nostril; this does not require more than a gentle touch.

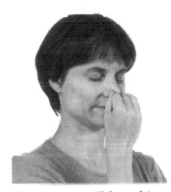

Alternate nostril breathing
(*nadi shodhanam*)

5. To begin the practice, gently close one nostril and exhale smoothly and completely through the other.

6. At the end of the exhalation, following the pattern of the variation you have chosen, inhale smoothly and completely. The duration of the inhalation and exhalation should be equal and there should be no sense of forcing your breath.

7. Continue exhaling and inhaling until you have completed one full round of the variation you have chosen. Then

breathe deeply and smoothly through both nostrils.

After you have worked with your chosen variation and achieved the ability to keep your exhalations and inhalations smooth, even, and noiseless, you will notice that the length of your breath tends to increase. Allow yourself to progress by letting the process become slower, smoother, and more consciously focused. When you can do that, you are ready for the next level.

Intermediate level of alternate nostril breathing

At the intermediate level, students should practice three rounds of *nadi shodhanam*, taking three breaths through both nostrils at the end of each round to rest and recover the natural internal rhythm of breathing. More than three breaths may be taken, if needed. (Note: When practicing three rounds in one sitting, the second of the three rounds begins with the opposite nostril, and the pattern of alternation is therefore the reverse of rounds one and three.)

As you progress in this practice you will want to give it more time and attention. Always keep the breath smooth and even. Do not force yourself to go beyond what is comfortable. There should not be any need to gasp or force the breath. Your goal is to achieve a subtle, smooth serenity in the breath.

Both two-to-one breathing and *nadi shodhanam* can be practiced twice a day, and other breathing practices can also be done after completing hatha yoga postures. However, breath retention should be done only under the supervision of a competent guide who has practiced it and who trains the student in the use of bandhas and mudras. Otherwise a disturbance in your vital force can create breathing disorders that are injurious for the heart, brain, and other systems.

There are numerous breathing exercises; just a few of the subtle practices have been explained here to help students attain a meditative state in which the breath flows freely in both nostrils. This opening of the breath is called the awakening of sushumna, and it is important for the higher stages of meditation. When sushumna is awakened, a particular clarity is realized, and the mind does not roam around but remains in a state of joy. Such a joyful mind is fit for meditation and attains a state of tranquility.

Chapter Six

A Program for Progress in Meditation

THIS PROGRAM FOR PROGRESS in meditation is the result of thorough examination and experimentation by the tradition of the sages. Many sincere students of meditation have experienced its benefits. If you really want to attain the highest state of meditation, you should commit yourself to following this system, which is simple.

- Learn to sit at the same time every day, and allow this to become a habit.
- Develop a good sitting posture for meditation. There are only a few postures that are appropriate for meditation. These include the easy pose, the auspicious pose, and the accomplished pose. Choose one pose and regularly practice that same position for meditation. Your body will adjust accordingly.

Guidelines and Goals for the First Month

The first one or two months should be devoted to attaining a still, comfortable posture. A meditative posture should be steady and comfortable. Steadiness of posture means that you are able to sit still and can keep the head, neck, and trunk aligned. Allowing the posture to become comfortable means that you are not uneasy or disturbed in any way. The cushion you use as a meditation seat should be neither too high nor too hard, and it should never be spongy or unstable.

For the first month, you may use the support of a wall to help you tell whether you are keeping your head, neck, and trunk in a straight line. After that, learn to sit independently of any external support. A good meditation seat can be made from a wooden plank or board covered with two blankets that are folded into quarters.

At the first level of practice, obstacles may arise in several dimensions. First, the body may shake, perspire, or become numb. Next, the subtler muscles, such as the cheeks or eyes, may twitch. You should learn to ignore all this. At first the body rebels when you try to discipline it. If your throat gets dry while you are doing meditation, you can take a few sips of water. In certain cases, you may notice that there is excess saliva in your mouth. Both of these symptoms may be due to overeating or consuming unhealthy food.

When you begin to sit in meditation, you should not try to sit for a long time. To start, 15 to 20 minutes will be sufficient. Every third day you can expand your practice by 3 minutes. Gradually, when your posture becomes steady, the time will extend itself. Developing a still, steady posture will bring you great joy. Discomfort is not a good sign; massage your toes, legs, and thighs when you get up from your meditation seat.

Pray to the Lord that your meditation will continue to become better, that you will remain motivated to sit in meditation, and that you look forward to your meditation time with great desire. But remember that you are praying to the Lord of Life, who is seated in the inner chamber of your own being. This sort of prayer strengthens your awareness. Do not pray for anything else except to strengthen your meditation. Selfish prayers feed the ego and make the aspirant weak and dependent. Prayer should be God-centered, not ego-centered.

Exercise 1

As you begin your meditation, survey your body mentally. Check to see that your eyes are gently closed, your teeth are gently touching, your lips are sealed, and your hands are placed lightly on your knees (or as near your knees as you can comfortably reach without slouching forward).

Complete this survey of your body systematically, from the crown of the head downward. In the forehead, let there be no tension; in the cheeks and jaw, no tension; in the neck and shoulders, no tension. From the arms to the fingertips there should be no tension.

Mentally return to your shoulders, allowing no tension. Let there be no tension in the chest. While your attention is at the chest, inhale and exhale within your comfortable capacity. This will help you relax your body. Take several deep breaths through your nostrils and mentally surrender any tension. Do not make suggestions to your body, but rather observe it and allow any tension to subside. Let your attention move on to the abdominal area. Survey the pelvic area, the hips, thighs, knees, calves, ankles, and feet.

Now inhale and exhale at least 5 to 10 times. Visualize your body and again systematically come back through the body in the reverse order, returning to the crown of your head. Survey your body thoroughly; if you find that a certain part of the body has any aches or pain, gently ask your mind to go to that spot to heal the ache. The mind definitely has the inner capacity to correct such discomforts. Do not doubt that.

Understanding the Mind

The mind is the master of the body, breath, and senses, for it is charged with the power of the center of consciousness, the individual soul. All our thinking processes, emotional power, capacity for analysis, and the functioning of the different modifications of the mind are due to the power of the innermost soul. One simply has to become aware of this fact, that the mind is in direct control of the senses, breath, and body. It is the mind that influences the senses and causes them to function in the external world. It is the mind that desires to perceive the world through the senses and to conceptualize and categorize those sensory perceptions. The mind stores its impressions in the unconscious, the storehouse of merits and demerits, and then recalls them whenever it needs them.

All *sadhanas* (spiritual practices, techniques, and disciplines) are actually meant to train the mind. And the foremost part of the training is to make the mind aware of that reality which lies beyond the mind: the immortal soul. The mind is a separate, individual entity, but it does not have a separate existence. It exists only because of the existence of the soul.

The mind is the finest instrument we possess. If it is understood well, the mind can be helpful in our sadhana. However, if the mind is not well-ordered and disciplined, it can distract us from our goals and dissipate all our potentials. Anything within the domain of the mind can be healed by the mind, once we know our deeper nature. When we become aware of our inner self, we can consciously heal, or prevent the occurrence of, many diseases.

There are four distinct functions of the mind: *manas*, *buddhi*, *ahamkara*, and *chitta*. These four should be understood and their functioning should be coordinated. Manas is the lower mind, through which we interact with the external world and take in sensory impressions and data. Manas also has the tendency to doubt and question, which can cause difficulties if this tendency becomes excessive.

Buddhi is the higher aspect of the mind, the doorway to inner wisdom. It has the capacity to decide, judge, and make cognitive discriminations and differentiations. It can determine the wiser of two courses of action, if it functions clearly and if manas will accept its guidance.

Ahamkara is the sense of "I-ness," the individual ego, which feels itself to be a distinct, separate entity. It provides us with our sense of identity, but also creates feelings of separation, pain, and alienation.

Chitta is the memory bank which stores our impressions and experiences. While it can be useful, chitta can also cause difficulties if it is not coordinated with the other functions. These four functions are described in greater detail in *The Art of Joyful Living*.

Just as aspirants should care for and pay attention to these different functions of the mind (manas, chitta, buddhi, and ahamkara), which have different abilities and duties, so also should they take care of their external behavior, so that they do not acquire the diseases transmitted through unhealthy food, sex, or imbalanced ways of living.

Cleanliness is valuable, but we should not become obsessive about it, because in order to function effectively, the immune system also requires a healthy mind. Purity of mind is achieved by ridding ourselves of negative, passive, and slothful mental tendencies. Such a healthy mind acquires self-confidence, and then buddhi can better discriminate and decide things on time.

To establish coordination among the various faculties of the mind, we have to learn to watch how the mind functions through our actions and speech, and at the same time observe the thinking process itself. Ignorance is the mother of all disease, discomfort, pain, and misery. A purified, quiet, and serene mind is positive and healthy. The process of meditation helps the mind remain a useful and constructive instrument.

A clear mind, which has been purified and trained to become one-pointed, can in many cases bring about healing. Self-healing is one of the natural physical capabilities of every person's mind. For example, suppose you are peeling an apple and cut your finger, and it begins to bleed. You'll notice that the cells of the body act as if they have a kind of understanding, and take immediate action at the site of the cut to stop the bleeding and protect the injured cells. In time, depending on the condition of the body's immune system, the body heals itself. But in a body whose mental and emotional processes are not coordinated, excessive cell activity may occur, which may even eventually create a growth. Due to such a lack of coordination and balance at a subtle level of mental functioning, diseases may arise and disturb our sadhana.

I believe that if we become emotionally attached to the external objects of the world, and remain unable to unfold our highest potential, then life is incomplete and we become victims of discontent and dissatisfaction. Therefore we should apply all our present resources to make the body, breath, senses, and mind healthy tools, so that sadhana is facilitated.

When you attain a state of meditation in which the body has become perfectly still and quiet, and doesn't move, shake, tremble, or twitch, then there is a feeling of unusual joy that is quite different from the other joys of worldly experience. Then you can begin to watch your breath, and enter the next stage of meditation.

Remember that practicing breath awareness is vital for meditation. Observe your breathing to see if you notice any problems with the four common faults we discussed earlier: jerkiness, shallowness, noise, or extended pauses. The body should be still, with the head, neck, and trunk aligned, so that your breathing can flow smoothly.

Practice for the Second Month

In the second month, you can extend your practice as follows.

After you have done your stretching and limbering exercises, then do your breathing exercises. To relax the gross muscles, physical exercises are helpful, but to create a deeper level of relaxation in the subtle muscles and nervous system, breathing exercises are even more useful. Alternate nostril breathing and even breathing are beneficial preparatory

practices, but during meditation itself, the only exercise recommended is breath awareness. Breath is one of the great
focal points of the mind. The mind and the breath are in-
separable associates. It is easy and natural for the mind to
focus on the breath.

As we said earlier, for the first month the aspirant should
focus the mind on the flow of the breath, watching and observing one's inhalations and exhalations, and seeking to remove the four main problems with the breath. In the next step
of breathing practice, the mind should be carefully focused on
the exercise described below.

Exercise 2

This will be a delightful experience, but remember that
you will experience this pleasant state only if you first learn
to make the posture steady, still, and comfortable, so that
your body will not distract you from the inner delight of this
breathing technique. This particular exercise is subtle; it is
more advanced and refined than the other experiences you
have had with breath awareness. It has been the focus of experiments done for thousands of years by a line of sages and
teachers.

Inhale as though you are breathing from the base of the
spine to the crown of the head, without creating any disturbances in the breath. Exhale as though you are exhaling
from the top of the head to the base of the spine. It will be
helpful if you can visualize three cords in the spine: in the
center, the channel physiologists call the *centralis canalis,*
and on the sides, the subtle channels yogis call *ida* and *pingala,* two of the main *nadis* described earlier.

Inhale and exhale through the centralis canalis, which is
an extremely fine milky-white tube. Feel the subtle current

of energy that flows between the medulla oblongata (at the base of the brain) and the pelvic plexus. Observe your mind and see how many times it becomes distracted. The moment the mind is distracted, you will find that there is a slight jerk or irregularity in the breath. During this practice it is recommended that you continue the gentle flow of the breath without jerks, noise, shallowness, or extended pauses.

After you inhale and exhale with awareness of the spine, become aware of the breath as it comes and goes through the nostrils. You may notice that one nostril seems blocked and the other may seem more open. You can easily inhale through one but not the other. In such cases, pay attention to the blocked nostril, and you may be surprised to notice that in a few moments' time, the blocked nostril opens.

For example, you might first pay attention to the right nostril. When it opens and becomes easy to breathe through, then pay attention to the other nostril, in order to open it simultaneously. If you practice this systematically, it will not take much time to develop control over the flow of the breath.

The breath and mind are twin laws of life. They are close to each other and easily influence each other. Although they have a separate existence, they register each other's influence. Try to establish the awareness that the flow of your breath can be directed by your conscious will, through the simple attention of your mind. Soon you will find that the moment your thoughts change, your breath also shifts.

After experimenting with the subtle electrical potentials associated with both nostrils, the sages discovered that these two aspects of breath have different natures. Breathing through the left side has a cooling effect, while breathing through the right side has a warming effect.

According to this advanced science of breath, when you notice that one nostril is more active, one of the *tattvas* (subtle elements) is active and becomes prominent, which creates a disturbance in the mind. This is what causes the alteration in the flow of your breath. The tattvas are affected by the manner in which the breath flows through the left and right nostrils, and your breath is affected by the predominant tattva. However, once you gain control over the breath, it can also give you control over the shifts in the tattvas, according to your level of discrimination and depth of concentration as a student of meditation. This is a profound science discussed in much greater detail in *Path of Fire and Light*.

Sushumna awakening

Now let us go on to the next step, the process of making the mind calm and joyous, so that it experiences delight in practicing meditation. This method is called sushumna awakening. The aspirant who has the patience to proceed according to this program will surely benefit. Those who are "economy readers" will probably read through this description without ever practicing it, and they will gain only a glimpse of this process. May God bless them and hopefully someday they will also walk on this path of light.

To begin the process of sushumna awakening, the meditator focuses the mind on the breath as it is felt between the two nostrils. Mind you, this does not mean to visually focus on the top of the nostrils or the tip of the nose; it is not *trataka* (gazing with the eyes). The goal is to focus awareness on the flow of the breath, at the bridge between the nostrils, just above the upper lip. When you focus your mind here, you will soon discover that both nostrils begin to flow freely. This is called *sandhya,* the wedding of the sun and moon, the union between pingala and ida. This is a delightful time in which neither worry, fear, nor other negative thoughts can distract the mind. However, it is important to realize that, because students do not have much experience in creating this state, it usually doesn't last long and is difficult to maintain for any length of time.

When you regularly focus the mind on the center between the two nostrils, morning and evening, you will find that the mind easily attains a state of joy. Then you feel eager to enter this state again and look forward to your meditation all day. When both nostrils flow freely, it means that you are inhaling and exhaling through both nostrils simultaneously, which is the sign of sushumna awakening. Once this experience can be maintained for five minutes, you have crossed a great barrier, and your mind has attained the beginning of one-pointedness. Now your mind starts to focus inward. Two to three months should be devoted to this *kriya* (special practice).

The Conscious Mind

The conscious mind is that part of the mind which functions during the waking state. It is merely a small fragment of the totality of the mind. Our educational system— whether at home, in school, or in the colleges and universities—has no systematic program that teaches us how to really understand and become aware of the whole of the mind, especially the unconscious mind. That tiny fraction of the mind that is cultivated by our educational system, from childhood onward, is merely the conscious mind.

The conscious mind relies on ten senses to collect data

from the external world. These consist of five subtle cognitive senses (sight, hearing, taste, smell, and touch) and five gross active senses (the hands, feet, power of speech, and organs of reproduction and elimination).

Most of us know only a little about how to educate the conscious aspect of our mind. The sages, however, with the assistance of deeper meditative methods, learned to dive deeply into the inner recesses of the unconscious and to make use of its capacities in an orderly way. These great ones are able to accomplish this with a simple, systematic method of meditation. Sadly, most human beings operate at a level of awareness barely above the level of the brute, because they don't know how to gain access into the deeper aspects of the mind. That is why we aren't aware of the inner treasures hidden in our deeper personalities.

There are many obstacles to overcome in order to help the conscious mind understand itself. The mind usually remains clouded, confused, and undisciplined, focused almost exclusively on objects in the external world, where everything seems to move and change. Because the mind itself is confused, even learning how to accurately perceive and assess objects and events in the external world is a serious problem for many people. However, those who are meditators learn to purify the mind and make it one-pointed. For them, it becomes possible to collect sense data exactly as they are. Such people see things clearly, rather than in the usual distorted or distracted fashion.

With the help of meditation, the conscious mind can be trained to form a new habit. The personality can be transformed when you learn to let go of the unhelpful, habitual thoughts arising in the conscious mind. Learn to witness your thoughts and practice remaining undisturbed, unaffected, and uninvolved in the scenes, feelings, concepts, and memories passing by in your mental train. Another three to four months of regular meditative practice will allow you enough time to learn to deal with the conscious aspect of the mind.

Sometimes people feel that they already have control over their mind, but that isn't usually true, because even if they can control their conscious mind, they cannot control the unknown unconscious mind, which is powerful and extensive. The unconscious is a vast reservoir of the impressions resulting from our deeds, actions, desires, and emotions. These latent levels of the mind remain a mystery to the average person. Even when the conscious mind has seemingly become calm, a single impression (such as a memory) that arises from the unconscious can suddenly disturb the mind, exactly the way a pebble's splash disturbs the smooth surface of a lake.

Human emotion is an immense power, which usually operates below the surface of the lake of mind, like a shark swimming under water. If that emotion is not guided, it can contaminate the whole lake. In this endeavor you need to learn to be patient with yourself. To be afraid to try to examine your thought process is a serious mistake to make. You should examine all your fears, and then you will find that most of them are imaginary and irrational. From this point you then begin the process of contemplation with analysis. Gradually you will acquire the ability to inspect your thinking process while remaining undisturbed. Such a mind attains clarity and is then prepared to attain samadhi. There are many levels of samadhi, which is a state of deep, absorbed meditation. When you can focus your mind for ten minutes without any disturbance, you have nearly attained this goal.

All human beings who are aware of the underlying reality of life, and who have already examined the joys and pleasures of the world and found them wanting, will realize that they cannot remain content or truly satisfied without practicing meditation. Meditation creates the highest of all joys. Meditation creates fearlessness.

The final step of meditation is to remain in silence. This silence cannot be described; it is inexplicable. This silence opens the door to intuitive knowledge, and then the past, present, and future are revealed to the student.

Once upon a time, a student of meditation went to see a sage. The student began discussing philosophical concepts, such as the nature of God, but the sage didn't say anything. The aspirant talked on and on and asked many probing questions, but still the sage kept still. Finally, in frustration, the aspirant asked why the sage wouldn't answer his questions. Then the sage smiled and said gently, "I have been answering, but you are not listening: God is silence."

In the course of my search and study in the Himalayas and other parts of India, I met a fortunate few who enjoyed this deep state of silence and also helped those who are prepared to meditate. Beyond body, breath, and mind lies this silence. From silence emanate peace, happiness, and bliss. Meditators make that silence their personal abode. That is the final goal of meditation.

QUESTIONS AND ANSWERS ON THE PRACTICE OF MEDITATION

Q: Why isn't "meditation music" considered helpful in deepening meditation?

A: Music is an external stimulus, which takes your sensory system and mind in the direction of external awareness, rather than toward the inward focus of meditation. Concentration on some pleasant, external stimulus—such as a rose or soft music—can be quite soothing, but it doesn't lead you in the direction of the highest state of consciousness within. Enjoy music at other times, but do not confuse this with meditation.

Q: What about using incense or candles? Are they necessary or helpful?

A: For the same reason, burning incense while meditating isn't recommended, because the scent or smoke can be a distraction. If you wish, burn a little incense before you meditate to establish a pleasant atmosphere, but we recommend that you put the incense out when you begin to meditate.

Candles that flicker can also be quite a distraction, even though your eyes are gently closed. If you can obtain a good quality, nonflickering candle, you'll find it less bothersome, but again, since your focus is not meant to be on the candle, an external light is not essential.

Q: There seem to be many different meditative traditions and techniques. What accounts for these differences? How do I know which technique is best for me?

A: All authentic meditative traditions seek to help students know their own innermost nature. These seemingly different techniques can be compared to many different paths up a mountain. Along the paths the view may differ, but from the mountaintop the ultimate experience is the same.

Some techniques of meditation use mantras (as discussed in this book), while other traditions use different practices, often involving focusing on the breath. Whatever practice you choose, it is important that you do it regularly and conscientiously. Different techniques are appropriate for different students, who may have varying personalities, inclinations, and capacities. Learn one method, apply it consistently over time, and observe what response you seem to be having to the practice.

The practice of meditation using breath awareness alone is not sufficient, because the aspirant should learn to go beyond the conscious and even the unconscious mind. Some traditions lead students beyond them, while other methods are limited to breath awareness alone. It is essential to develop a comfortable, still posture, and then to become aware of the breath, but a human being is also a thinking being, and cannot ignore dealing with the various levels of the mind. Therefore a technique that leads aspirants beyond all the levels of the mind is a higher method of meditation. We do not condemn other meditation techniques, but some are complete and some are incomplete.

Eventually aspirants have to become aware of their essential nature, the source of consciousness, from which consciousness flows through various degrees and grades. The center of consciousness lies beyond the body, senses, breath, and mind. Therefore a method that is comprehensive and leads to the removal of all barriers to the experience of one's innermost being is the best method.

Q: Not only are there many different techniques, but there are different paths of yoga, such as the path of devotion and the path of action. Which should I follow?

A: There are many diverse paths, but the goal is only one. The path in which you find inner satisfaction is your own path. Become aware of what path you feel is right for you.

Q: Should I use an alarm clock to time my meditation?

A: From the beginning you should learn to strengthen your *sankalpa shakti* (power of will) by resolving that you will rise on time and meditate for 10, 15, or 20 minutes. The mind is the greatest of all timekeepers, and as you progress, you will find that the mind wakes you up for your meditation. Nothing external is really needed when you have decided that you want to awaken and meditate at a particular time.

Generally it's not necessary to use an alarm clock to time the meditation itself, since in meditation, unlike the state of sleep, you will not lose consciousness of the passage of time. It's also rather unpleasant to end a tranquil meditation with the jarring tone of an alarm clock. If you're concerned about the time, keep a clock within view so you can check the time, or better still, try to set up your meditation session so that you don't feel so much time pressure. Meditate earlier in the morning, or in the evening when there are no more duties or responsibilities awaiting you.

Q: What do I do if my legs begin to hurt or fall asleep?

A: This often happens when the aspirant does not do enough physical exercise, but if you begin to do stretching exercises before and after meditation, you will notice a difference after a few days. If you still experience discomfort, or if your feet fall asleep, stretch out your legs and shift position for a few minutes. You can massage or stretch your muscles and then, when your legs feel comfortable, resume your original position. You will find that the length of time you can sit comfortably will gradually increase as you form a habit of sitting regularly, and in a few months the body will not feel the way it did in the beginning.

Most modern people don't spend much time sitting on the floor, so initially some postures may be uncomfortable. However, you will probably find that as you become accustomed to your meditation posture, it feels increasingly natural. While it is commonplace for the body to have some initial difficulty adjusting to sitting on the floor (or any other new exercise), remember that you should never push your body to the point of pain. Physical exercise before and after the practice of meditation is important in helping to maintain good blood circulation.

Q: Sometimes my meditation is good and sometimes it is full of disturbances. How can I deal with this situation?

A: When your mind remains preoccupied by worldly concerns and desires, it interferes with your experience during meditation. In such cases, you should cultivate a firm determination to let go of all the thoughts that are coming forward in the mind asking for your attention. Therefore, before you sit in meditation, it is important to have a determined mind and to elevate your awareness by doing breath awareness. Decide not to be disturbed no matter what type of thoughts come into the conscious mind from the storehouse of merits and demerits, the unconscious mind. When you learn to witness your thinking process without becoming involved with its images, feelings, thoughts, and interests, then no thoughts—good or bad, helpful or unhelpful—can disturb you.

Q: Sometimes the body itches, the head tilts to one side, or other symptoms—such as yawning, spontaneous tearing of the eyes, or the need to swallow—occur. What is the correct way of dealing with these disturbances?

A: Such disturbances occur during the preliminary stages of meditation. If one does not overeat, learns to keep the mind free from preoccupations, and observes the body, these things can be checked easily.

Q: Why do I feel afraid during meditation?

A: This problem often occurs in those who have avoided becoming aware of certain desires and suppressed thoughts, as well as those who wish to escape from self-awareness, not wanting to analyze or understand their thinking process.

Actually a student is always safe during meditation, because the closer one is to the innermost, immortal reality, the safer one becomes. It is true that in meditation, hidden motivations and repressed feelings do become conscious, but the aspirant should cultivate inner strength and allow these things to come to awareness, and then learn to let go of them so they do not continue to distract the mind. Sincere effort and practicing meditation consistently and regularly, with firm determination, eventually help the student overcome such hurdles.

Q: What is japa? How does it help to deepen meditation?

A: Japa is the continuous mental repetition of one's mantra. It is a helpful tool for keeping the mind focused on maintaining awareness of the center of consciousness. One can do japa all the time, in all situations and conditions. One of the best ways of doing japa is the silent technique of reciting the mantra without moving one's tongue. The mind has a habit of always thinking of and obsessing about both the desirable and undesirable objects or events of the world. Keeping the mind busy doing japa is a useful accomplishment which counteracts this tendency. When japa becomes *ajapa japa* (spontaneous and effortless, going on by itself), it creates inner comfort, joy, peace, and happiness. If japa is done with feeling, and not mere mechanical repetition, it helps the student in attaining *mahabhava* (ecstasy).

In all spiritual traditions of the world, some form of japa is recommended. It is one of the great supports and aids for an aspirant of meditation. Japa can be done using a *mala*, which is a set of beads much like a rosary, or it can be done only mentally. If you use a mala, you move one bead each time you repeat the mantra.

Q: What is the difference between meditation and mental japa?

A: Japa leads the meditator like a constant companion,

helping the meditator cross all the intervening barriers to reach a state of silence. Silence is the greatest of all attainments. It is an experience in which one remains fully conscious and aware of the inner reality or Self, which is the Self of all, the universal truth.

Q: Do diet and sexual activity affect one's meditation?

A: Of course these factors affect meditation, so the mind should not be encouraged to roam and obsess in sexual grooves all the time. Sex is a biological and emotional necessity to a certain age, although this appetite should be regulated. This should not become the most prominent and dominating purpose of one's life.

As far as food is concerned, simple, fresh, nutritious food that is not overcooked is best for the student of meditation. However, even though foods that are rich in nutrients are most healthy, overeating is neither healthy nor conducive to meditation. Meditation should not be done either when one is hungry or just after one has eaten.

Q: How do I know when I need a teacher and how do I find one?

A: When aspirants begin to examine the momentary and transitory nature of the objects of the external world, they find they are no longer fully satisfied with them. They begin questioning the purpose of life and then try to understand their own internal states. Often, such students study the sayings of the sages. It is during this period of seeking that students find they need a guide. There is an ancient saying—which is true—that when a student has a burning desire to know the innermost truth, is sincerely searching, and is prepared, then the teacher appears.

All aspirants should know that an authentic teacher is always selfless and knows the state of mind of the aspirant and guides them accordingly. Do not search for a teacher, but prepare yourself first, and your teacher will come. Those teachers who are selfish and dominating or who exploit their students can never really guide anyone. Teachers who are selfless, experienced, and who practice meditation know whether aspirants are actually prepared to tread the path. It is true that a competent teacher is a gift of grace from God.

I advise seekers not to run here and there in search of teachers, but rather to prepare themselves by watching their own mind, action, and speech, for there is a teacher within everyone, and that is their own conscience. If we ignore our inner teacher, then a teacher outside will be of no use to us. Learning to listen to one's conscience is a great preparation for the path of spirituality.

Sometimes the ego comes forward and misguides us. The mind is a magician which can play many tricks, but the sincere aspirant will learn to recognize when the inner guidance received comes from their conscience or from a deluded or egotistic part of their personality. I advise students to pray to the mighty Self within, for heartfelt prayers are always answered.

Q: How do students know that they are progressing?

A: Progressing on the path of spirituality is not like progressing in the external world. On the inner path, progressing means developing a peaceful and joyous mind. The student does not feel agitated or excited. This inner experience is a sufficient indication of the progress of the aspirant. The aspirant is also bound to meet others on the path of spirituality who share similar goals, for the law of nature is that similar attracts similar.

Q: Can meditation cure emotional problems?

A: Meditation is the highest of all therapies, provided it is practiced systematically. Gradually aspirants learn to deal with their problems, fears, and habit patterns. Every human being has the capacity to advance and is fully equipped to deal even with gigantic problems, provided they follow their path with firm determination and sincerity. If when your human efforts are exhausted you still do not find peace within, then surrender yourself to the Self of all, the Lord of Life. Such self-surrender is the highest of all methods.

Q: Are there any dangers in practicing meditation?

A: Meditation is not at all dangerous, but if we are not prepared, then sitting with closed eyes and hallucinating is a sheer waste of time and energy. We should understand the whole method and gradually train ourselves to be "insiders." Most of us are taught to learn, watch, and verify things only in the external world. Learning to look, find, and see within is an entirely different path. Therefore learning to practice meditation systematically is useful.

Many teachers claim that their methods are a shortcut, and that other methods are lengthy. There is no such thing as a shortcut or a lengthy process; the path depends entirely on the student's capacity, sincerity, and determination. Do not be swayed by such propaganda, publicity, or promotions. Work with yourself.

Q: What are the symptoms of deepening meditation?

A: Meditation makes the mind one-pointed and inward. When you have learned to arrange your worldly duties so that they don't create any obstacles, and when you practice meditation regularly and punctually, then you will find it rewarding in a special way. The mind becomes penetrating and one-pointed, and starts to fathom the subtler dimensions of life. These are the symptoms of deepening meditation.

Q: How does one develop a feeling for the mantra?

A: In the beginning, simply follow the technique of mantra repetition. Later on, as this habit becomes a part of your life, you start to experience joy. You actually love your habits, and when the japa becomes an irreplaceable habit of your life, you feel attracted to and delighted by the mantra.

Q: What is the final outcome of meditation? What can we expect?

A: The books all say that the final outcome is the attainment of samadhi. There are various types of samadhi, but I can tell you that a meditator is fully capable of attaining the highest state of wisdom, in which the mind cannot and does not pose any questions, because all questions are answered and all problems are resolved. This delightful state of mind brings tranquility in the external world and permanent peace within. Such meditators remain aware of truth at every moment and become fearless, for they remember the Lord of Life in every breath, and live in the world unaffected by worldly turmoil.

Q: How long will it take a sincere student to attain the final goal?

A: This depends on the quality of the students' internal states and the intensity of their determination, as well as the punctuality and regularity they maintain in meditation practice. Some students become excited and emotional about wanting to attain the highest state. They practice enthusiastically for a few days, but then their interest wanes and they stop practicing. However, those who persevere, practicing their meditation with regularity and full determination, surely attain the highest wisdom in a short time. Aspirants have many fantasies, desires for inner experiences, and expectations of miracles, but when they understand that these are not helpful, then they abandon them and step beyond the mire of delusion, treading the path of light.

RECOMMENDATIONS FOR FURTHER STUDY

The following will be especially helpful in advancing your understanding and practice of meditation:

The Art of Joyful Living by Swami Rama

Creative Use of Emotion by Swami Rama

Inner Quest by Pandit Rajmani Tigunait, Ph.D.

Living with the Himalayan Masters by Swami Rama

Path of Fire and Light, Volumes I and II by Swami Rama

The Power of Mantra and the Mystery of Initiation by Pandit Rajmani Tigunait, Ph.D.

The Royal Path: Practical Lessons on Yoga by Swami Rama (formerly *Lectures on Yoga*)

Science of Breath by Swami Rama, Rudolph Ballentine, M.D., and Alan Hymes, M.D.

Superconscious Meditation by Usharbudh Arya, D.Litt.

Transition to Vegetarianism by Rudolph Ballentine, M.D.

Yoga: Mastering the Basics by Sandra Anderson and Rolf Sovik, Psy.D.

You may also find several relaxation and meditation tapes to be useful, including:

Guided Meditation for Beginners
A Guide to Intermediate Meditation
First Step Toward Advanced Meditation
Learn to Meditate
31 and 61 Points

These and other books and tapes on meditation are available from the Himalayan Institute Press. For a catalog or further information, call 800-822-4547 or 717-253-5551, e-mail: hibooks@epix.net, or fax: 717-251-7812.

For students interested in practicing japa, a Japa Kit containing full instructions and a mala (yoga rosary) is also available.

APPENDIX A:
RELAXATION EXERCISES

Tension/Relaxation Exercise

This exercise is done for three minutes at the beginning of your hatha yoga session. It can be practiced for several weeks or until your body and mind have started letting go of tension through the practice of hatha postures, breathing exercises, and meditation.

Technique

Lie in the corpse posture, relaxed and breathing evenly.

Tense all the muscles of the face, pulling them toward the tip of the nose. Then release the tension and relax.

Gently close the eyes and keep them closed throughout the rest of the exercise.

Gently roll the head from side to side several times.

Pull the shoulders forward. Gently release and relax.

Tense the right arm in a subtle manner, without making a fist or lifting the arm off the floor. Do not focus exclusively on tensing only the external muscles; take your mind deeper within the muscle structure. Then release the tension and relax.

Repeat with the left arm.

Tense the hips and the buttocks. Then release the tension and relax.

Tense the right leg in the same manner that you tensed the right arm. Then release the tension and relax.

Repeat with the left leg.

Starting at the toes, relax the body from the toes through the legs, torso, arms, neck, and head.

Complete Relaxation Exercise

Before meditating it is beneficial to do a concentrated relaxation exercise. There are many such techniques. The one described here relaxes the skeletal muscles, eliminates any fatigue or strain following the hatha yoga postures, and energizes both the mind and the body. During this exercise, keep your mind alert and concentrated on your breath as you progressively relax your muscles.

In the beginning you should practice this technique for only ten minutes, because beyond that time the mind usually begins to wander and you may find yourself drifting toward sleep.

Technique

Lie in the corpse posture with your eyes gently closed. Inhale and exhale through your nostrils slowly, smoothly, and deeply. There should be no noise, jerks, or pauses in your breath. Let your inhalations and exhalations flow naturally, without exertion, in one continuous movement. Keep the body still.

Mentally travel through your body and relax the top of the head, forehead, eyebrows, the space between your eyebrows, eyes, eyelids, cheeks, and nose. Then exhale and inhale completely four times, breathing diaphragmatically.

Exhaling, relax your mouth, jaw, chin, neck, shoulders, upper arms, lower arms, wrists, hands, fingers, and fingertips. Feel as if you are inhaling from your fingertips, up your arms, shoulders, and face to your nostrils, and then exhaling back to the fingertips. Then exhale and inhale completely four times.

Relax your fingertips, fingers, hands, wrists, lower arms, upper arms, shoulders, upper back, and chest. Concentrate at the center of the chest, and exhale and inhale completely four times.

Relax the stomach, abdomen, lower back, hips, thighs, knees, calves, ankles, feet, and toes.

Exhale as though your whole body is exhaling, and inhale as though your whole body is inhaling. Expel all your tension, worries, and anxieties. Inhale vital energy, peace, and relaxation. Exhale and inhale completely four times.

Relax your toes, feet, ankles, calves, thighs, knees, hips, lower back, abdomen, stomach, and chest. Concentrating at the center of the chest, exhale and inhale completely four times.

Relax your upper back, shoulders, upper arms, lower arms, wrists, hands, fingers, and fingertips. Then exhale and inhale completely four times.

Relax your fingertips, fingers, hands, wrists, lower arms, upper arms, shoulders, neck, chin, jaw, mouth, and nostrils. Then exhale and inhale completely four times.

Relax your cheeks, eyelids, eyes, eyebrows, the space between your eyebrows, forehead, and top of your head. Now, for 30 to 60 seconds, allow your mind to be aware of the calm and serene flow of your breath. Let your mind make a gentle, conscious effort to guide your breath so that it remains smooth, calm, and deep, without any noise or jerks.

Slowly and gently open your eyes. Stretch your body. Try to maintain this calm, peaceful feeling throughout the day.

Appendix B:
Breath Training

There are many breathing exercises designed to help beginning students. Here is a review of the basic practices leading to relaxed, diaphragmatic breathing in a meditative pose.

The Standing Complete Breath—a preparatory stretch

The standing complete breath helps in expanding the capacity of the lungs and is excellent for physical and mental energizing. During the exercise breathe through the nose, not the mouth. If possible, practice in front of an open window or outside in the fresh air.

When doing the exercise it may be helpful to picture a glass of water being filled and emptied. As the glass is being filled, the water level rises from bottom to top. When water in the glass is emptying, the water level descends from the top of the glass to the bottom. Similarly, as you inhale, imagine that the breath is filling your lungs to the top, and as you exhale, the lungs are emptied to the bottom.

Technique

Assume the simple standing posture.

Inhaling, slowly raise the arms to the sides, extending and

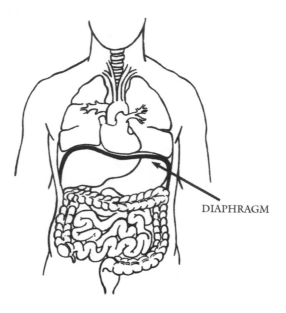

DIAPHRAGM

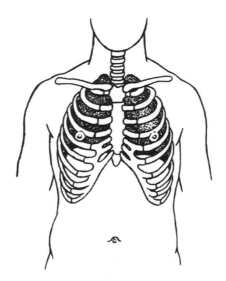

Location of the diaphragm in relation to
the ribs and internal organs.

lifting them gradually overhead until the palms are touching, in a prayer position. As you raise the arms, fill the lower lungs, then the middle lungs, and then the upper portion of the lungs.

Exhaling, slowly lower the arms back to the sides. You are emptying the upper portion of the lungs, then the middle of the lungs, and finally the lower lungs.

Repeat the exercise two to five more times.

Diaphragmatic Breathing

The training needed to learn diaphragmatic breathing can be accomplished in three steps. These steps are briefly summarized below, followed by exercises for practice.

1. Lying on the back in shavasana (the corpse pose)

Lying on the back, the rib cage is virtually motionless, while the navel area rises prominently with the inhalation and falls with the exhalation. This type of breathing is sometimes called "belly" breathing. It is not the final stage of diaphragmatic breathing, but it does help to eliminate the unhealthy habit of breathing with the chest and makes one aware of the effects of contracting the diaphragm. During this stage of practice you can begin to develop the various qualities of good breathing, making your breath deep, smooth, even, without sound, and without pause. To strengthen the diaphragm, practice sandbag breathing in this posture.

Technique

Lie on your back in shavasana (the corpse posture). Support your head and neck with a thin cushion. Rest your legs about twelve inches apart; place your arms a few inches from your torso, with palms turned up.

Close your eyes and let your body become still. Rest the muscles of your rib cage until the chest and ribs become almost motionless. Then begin to observe the flow of your breathing. Notice the rise and fall of your abdomen with each breath. Do not try to push the abdomen upward. Simply let it rise as your diaphragm contracts and descends naturally, creating the inhalation. As you exhale, observe the fall of your abdomen.

At the end of each phase of your breathing, relax and let the next phase begin. Each inhalation flows naturally into the exhalation without pause; each exhalation flows into the inhalation, again, without pause.

Let your breath become deep and smooth. Breathe without jerks and without "trying" hard to control the breath. Each inhalation and exhalation is approximately equal in length. In addition, as the breath becomes deeper and slower, let it flow without sound.

Finally, observe the breath over and over as if the body breathes and you are simply watching it. Let your mind relax as you watch the breath for an additional five minutes.

2. Lying on the stomach in the crocodile pose

Lying on the stomach in the crocodile posture, you will notice that the ribs at the lower sides of the rib cage are free to move with breathing. They expand with the inhalation and contract with the exhalation. When lying on the stomach, the back also rises and falls with each breath. By bringing awareness to the sides and back, in addition to the abdomen, this stage of breath training introduces a more complete feeling of the dynamics of diaphragmatic breathing.

Technique

Lie on your stomach. Fold your arms on the floor above your head, and place your forehead on your forearms. Your legs may be together, or apart—the toes turned in or out. Let your whole body rest.

Observe the flow of your breathing, feeling the rise and fall of your lower back with each breath. The back rises with inhalation and falls with exhalation.

Next observe the movement of the sides of the rib cage. The ribs expand with each inhalation and contract with the exhalation.

Finally, feel the abdomen press against the floor as you inhale and contract as you exhale.

Watch your body breathe, observing these movements around the entire lower part of your torso—the back, sides, and abdomen. Continue for an additional five minutes, letting your nervous system and mind relax as your watch the breath.

3. Sitting erect (in any meditation pose)

In an erect sitting pose the muscles of the abdomen and lower back are moderately active in order to maintain the posture. This affects the breathing. As in the crocodile posture, the front, sides, and back all expand with inhalation. The sideward expansion of the lower ribs is most noticeable, while the movement of the abdomen is somewhat less marked, and the back moves only slightly.

Technique

Sit erect in one of the seated meditation postures. Let your body rest and become still. Relax the muscles of the chest, lower back, and abdomen, while maintaining an erect posture.

Observe the flow of your breathing, feeling the lower torso expand with each inhalation and contract as you exhale. Notice how your breathing results in a quiet expansion of sides, front, and back—each balancing the role played by the other.

The abdominal movement is not nearly so prominent while sitting as while lying down. The movement of the sides is much more noticeable.

Continue to watch the breath for another five minutes, relaxing and learning to recognize the feel of diaphragmatic breathing in a sitting posture. During that time, let thoughts come and go while maintaining your awareness of the breath.

GLOSSARY

Ahamkara   Loosely translated as "ego." Together, manas, buddhi, chitta, and ahamkara comprise the four functions of the mind. It is through ahamkara that one identifies oneself with the objects of the world, feeling, for example, "I am this body." It refers to a faculty of mind through which pure consciousness falsely identifies itself with non-self, that is, the mind, physical body, and material objects.

Ajapa Japa   The constant spontaneous awareness of one's mantra.

Asana   Literally, "sitting," "position," or "posture." The fourth of the eight limbs of raja yoga, which emphasizes attainment of a steady and comfortable posture. It later evolved into the science of physical culture called hatha yoga in which the word means one of the systems of postures.

Atman   Pure consciousness, the true Self, the unchanging, eternal truth which is beyond the entire manifest world.

Aum (or Om)   A sound which represents the Absolute. According to the yogic scriptures called the Upanishads, the word *Aum* consists of three letters—A, U, and M—representing the waking, dreaming, and deep sleep states. After the word *Aum* is pronounced, there comes a moment of silence, which represents the absolute or transcendent reality beyond these three ordinary states of awareness. The highest of mantras, *Aum* is a symbol of the highest realization and knowledge.

Bandha   "Lock." An internal bodily constriction or contraction applied for the purpose of stopping or directing prana.

Bhava   Emotion, mood, devotional state of mind, feeling.

Buddhi   The mental faculty of the intellect. Buddhi has three main functions: it knows, evaluates, and makes decisions.

Chitta   The pool of the unconscious mind in which all the impressions gathered by the senses are deposited, and from the bottom of which they arise to create a constant stream of random thoughts and associations.

Dhyana   Meditation; a one-pointed state of mind that is not disturbed by any thought constructs.

Hatha Yoga   The science of physical health that developed out of the third limb of raja yoga—asana. It attempts, through physical postures and cleansing exercises, to prepare the student for higher practices in yoga.

Ida   One of the three principal energy channels flowing in the spinal cord. It controls the breath in the left nostril.

Japa   Repetition of one's mantra. Constant japa is an excellent technique for making the mind one-pointed. Japa as a practice is complete in itself, provided it is done with knowledge and full devotion.

Kundalini   The inner fire or fundamental life-energy. Kundalini in its dormant, coiled state resides at the base of the spine. By following a systematic discipline of pranayama, meditation, and mantra japa, one prepares oneself for kundalini awakening.

Kriya   Action, activity. Kriya yoga in this context means the path of action.

Mahabhava   The state of ecstasy.

Maitri Asana   Friendship pose, a meditative posture involving sitting on a chair or platform.

Manas   Mind. One of the inner mental instruments. It receives information from the external world with the help of the senses, and presents it to the higher faculty of intellect. This particular faculty is also characterized by doubt.

Mantra   A combination of syllables or words corresponding to a particular energy vibration. The student, when initiated by a qualified teacher, utilizes the mantra as his object for meditation. As he practices over a period of time, the mantra gradually leads his meditation deeper and deeper. Through constant mantra repetition, both during meditation and in active life, the power of the mantra and its inner significance will gradually unfold as its latent mental and spiritual energies are released.

Mudra   Certain bodily gestures, like the finger lock, that are used to deepen meditation.

Nadi   Energy channel; one of the subtle channels of the body.

Nadi Shodhanam   Literally, "purifying the nadis." A breathing exercise that purifies the nadis in preparation for the higher practices of pranayama. Also known as channel purification or alternate nostril breathing, it attempts to quiet the mind and regulate the breath by establishing a slow, even rhythm, without a pause between the inhalation and exhalation.

Om   See *Aum*.

Padmasana   The lotus posture. A seated posture for breathing exercises.

Patanjali   A sage who was the codifier of yoga science.

Pingala   One of the three nadis or energy channels running parallel to the spinal column. It controls the flow of breath in the right nostril. When this channel becomes active, one's behavior is characterized by rationality, activity, and energy.

Prana   The life-force. In the yogic tradition, prana is said to take ten forms, depending on its nature and function.

Pranayama   Voluntary control over the pranic force; the fourth rung of raja yoga. The science of gradually lengthening and controlling the physical breath in order to gain control over the movement of prana through the subtle body in higher stages of yogic practice.

Raja Yoga   Literally, "royal path." The eightfold path of yoga as described by Patanjali in the *Yoga Sutras*.

Sadhana   Practice, spiritual endeavor. Literally, "accomplishing" or "fulfilling." Sadhana is the word for a student's sincere efforts along a particular path of practice toward self-realization.

Samadhi   Spiritual absorption; the eighth rung of raja yoga. The tranquil state in which fluctuations of the mind no longer arise.

Samskaras   Subtle impressions left in the mind by past actions.

Sankalpa Shakti   The mental power of dynamic will or resolution.

Shanti   Peace.

Shavasana   The corpse posture. A posture involving lying on one's back for relaxation.

Siddhi   Accomplishment, perfection, achievement. In practicing yoga, as one progresses toward the center of consciousness, advanced human potentials may unfold which can be very attractive and distracting. The goal of yoga is not to become caught by these supernatural abilities, but to go beyond.

Siddhasana   The accomplished posture. A sitting posture used for breathing exercises and meditation.

Sukhasana   The easy posture. A sitting posture used for breathing exercises and meditation.

Sushumna   The central energy channel or nadi that runs along the spinal column from its base to the crown of the head. The goal of preliminary breathing exercises is to open this central channel so that both nostrils are flowing equally. Then the mind enters a joyful state in which it easily attains a deep state of meditation.

Swarodaya   The ancient science of breath through which the sages learned much about human functioning and subtler energies.

Swastikasana   The auspicious posture. A sitting posture used for breathing exercises and meditation.

Tattva   Element. There are five physical elements: earth, water, fire, air, and space, and numerous subtle elements.

Trataka   The practice of gazing in order to strengthen concentration.

Yoga   The word *yoga* is generated from the Sanskrit root *yuj*, which means union. It is the systematic application of certain practices with proven effects and benefits.

Yoga Sutras   A manual on raja yoga compiled by the sage Patanjali around 200 B.C. It describes the basic outline of yoga philosophy and practice.

About the Author

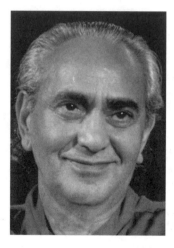

BORN IN 1925 in northern India, Swami Rama was raised from early childhood by a great Bengali yogi and saint who lived in the foothills of the Himalayas. In his youth he practiced the various disciplines of yoga science and philosophy in the traditional monasteries of the Himalayas and studied with many spiritual adepts, including Mahatma Gandhi, Sri Aurobindo, and Rabindranath Tagore. He also traveled to Tibet to study with his grandmaster.

He received his higher education at Bangalore, Prayaga, Varanasi, and Oxford University, England. At the age of twenty-four he became Shankaracharya of Karvirpitham in South India, the highest spiritual position in India. During this term he had a tremendous impact on the spiritual customs of that time: he dispensed with useless formalities and rituals, made it possible for all segments of society to worship in the temples, and encouraged the instruction of women in meditation. He renounced the dignity and prestige of this high office in 1952 to return to the Himalayas to intensify his yogic practices.

After completing an intense meditative practice in the cave monasteries, he emerged with the determination to serve humanity, particularly to bring the teachings of the East to the West. With the encouragement of his master, Swami Rama began his task by studying Western philosophy and psychology. He worked as a medical consultant in London and assisted in parapsychological research in Moscow. He then returned to India, where he established an ashram in Rishikesh. He completed his degree in homeopathy at the medical college in Darbhanga in 1960. He came to the United States in 1969, bringing his knowledge and wisdom to the West. His teachings combine Eastern spirituality with modern Western therapies.

Swami Rama was a freethinker, guided by his direct experience and inner wisdom, and he encouraged his students to be guided in the same way. He often told them, "I am a messenger, delivering the wisdom of the Himalayan sages of my tradition. My job is to introduce you to the teacher within."

Swami Rama came to America upon the invitation of Dr. Elmer Green of the Menninger Foundation of Topeka, Kansas, as a consultant in a research project investigating the voluntary control of involuntary states. He participated in experiments that helped to revolutionize scientific thinking about the relationship between body and mind, amazing scientists by his demonstrating, under laboratory conditions, precise conscious control of autonomic physical responses and mental functioning, feats previously thought to be impossible.

Swami Rama founded the Himalayan International Institute of Yoga Science and Philosophy, the Himalayan Institute Hospital Trust in India, and many centers thoughout the world. He is the author of numerous books on health, meditation, and the yogic scriptures. Swami Rama left his body in November 1996.

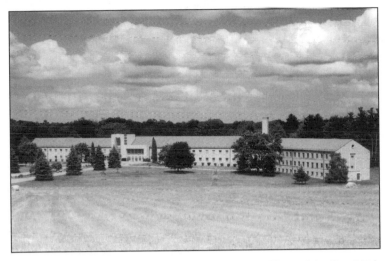

Main building of the international headquarters, Honesdale, Pa., USA

The Himalayan Institute

FOUNDED IN 1971 by Swami Rama, the Himalayan Institute has been dedicated to helping people grow physically, mentally, and spiritually by combining the best knowledge of both the East and the West. Institute programs emphasize holistic health, yoga, and meditation, but the Institute is much more than its programs.

Our international headquarters is located on a beautiful 400-acre campus in the rolling hills of the Pocono Mountains of northeastern Pennsylvania. The atmosphere here is one to foster growth, increased inner awareness, and calm. Our grounds provide a wonderfully peaceful and healthy setting for our seminars and extended programs.

Students from around the world join us here to attend programs in such diverse areas as hatha yoga, meditation, stress reduction, Ayurveda, nutrition, Eastern philosophy, psychology, and other subjects. Whether the programs are for weekend meditation retreats, week-long seminars on spirituality, months-long residential programs, or holistic health services, the attempt here is to provide an environment of gentle inner progress. We invite you to join with us in the ongoing process of personal growth and development.

The Institute is a nonprofit organization. Your membership in the Institute helps to support its programs. Please call or write for information on becoming a member.

Institute Programs, Services, and Facilities

All Institute programs share an emphasis on conscious holistic living and personal self-development. You may enjoy any of a number of diverse programs, including:

> Special weekend or extended seminars to teach skills and techniques for increasing your ability to be healthy and enjoy life
>
> Meditation retreats and advanced meditation instruction
>
> Vegetarian cooking and nutritional training
>
> Hatha yoga and exercise workshops
>
> Residential programs for self-development
>
> The Institute's Center for Health and Healing, which offers holistic health services and Ayurvedic Rejuvenation Programs.

The Institute publishes a *Quarterly Guide to Programs and Other Offerings,* which is free within the USA. To request a copy, or for further information, call 800-822-4547 or 717-253-5551, fax 717-253-9078, e-mail BQinfo@himalayaninstitute.org, or write the Himalayan Institute/RR 1, Box 400/Honesdale, PA 18431-9706 USA.

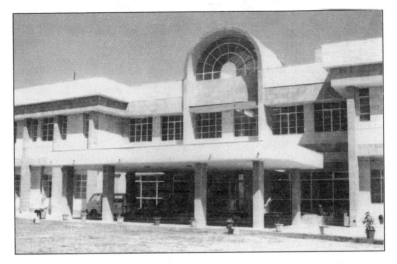

The main building of the hospital, outside Dehra Dun

Himalayan Institute Hospital and Medical City

A major aspect of the Institute's work around the world is its support of a comprehensive Medical City in the Garhwal region of the foothills of the Himalayas. A bold vision to bring medical services to 15 million mostly poor people who have little or no healthcare in northern India began modestly in 1989 with an outpatient program in Uttar Pradesh.

Today that vision has grown to include a fully operational, 500-bed, state-of-the-art hospital located between Dehra Dun and Rishikesh; a Medical College and nursing school, a combined therapy program that joins the best of modern, Western medicine and the time-tested wisdom of traditional methods of healthcare; a rural development program that has adopted more than 150 villages; and housing facilities for staff, students, and patients' relatives.

The project was conceived, designed, and led by Swami Rama, who was a native of this part of India. He always envisioned joining the best knowledge of the East and West. And that is what is occurring at this medical facility, 125 miles north of New Delhi.

Guided by the Himalayan Institute Hospital Trust, the umbrella body for the entire project, the hospital, medical city, and rural development program are considered models of healthcare for the whole of India and for medically under-served people worldwide.

Construction, expansion, and the fund-raising necessary to accomplish it all continues. The hospital is now one of the best-equipped hospitals in India, but more still needs to be done.

We welcome financial support to help with this and other projects. If you would like further information, please call our international headquarters in Honesdale, PA at 800-822-4547 or 717-253-5551, e-mail BMCinfo@himalayanin-stitute.org, fax 717-253-9078, or write RR 1, Box 400, Honesdale, PA 18431-9706 USA.

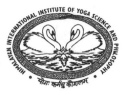

The Himalayan Institute Press

The Himalayan Institute Press has long been regarded as "The Resource for Holistic Living." We publish dozens of titles, as well as audio and video tapes, that offer practical methods for harmonious living and inner balance. Our approach addresses the whole person—body, mind, and spirit—integrating the latest scientific knowledge with ancient healing and self-development techniques.

As such, we offer a wide array of titles on physical and psychological health and well-being, spiritual growth through meditation and other yogic practices, and the means to stay inspired through reading sacred scriptures and ancient philosophical teachings.

Our sidelines include the Japa Kit for meditation practice, The Neti™ Pot, the ideal tool for sinus and allergy sufferers, and The Breath Pillow,™ a unique tool for learning health-supportive breathing—the diaphragmatic breath.

Subscriptions are available to a bimonthly magazine, *Yoga International*, which offers thought-provoking articles on all aspects of meditation and yoga, including yoga's sister science, Ayurveda.

For a free catalog call 800-822-4547 or 717-253-5551, e-mail hibooks@himalayaninstitute.org, or fax 717-251-7812.

Visit our Web site at www.himalayaninstitute.org.